A Visual History of HIV/AIDS

T0175653

The Face of AIDS film archive at Karolinska Institutet, Sweden, consists of more than 700 hours of unedited and edited footage, shot over a period of more than thirty years and all over the world by filmmaker and journalist Staffan Hildebrand. The material documents the HIV/AIDS pandemic and includes scenes from conferences and rallies, and interviews with activists, physicians, people with the infection, and researchers. It represents a global historical development from the early years of the AIDS crisis to a situation in which it is possible to live a normal life with the HIV virus. This volume brings together a range of academic perspectives – from media and film studies, medical history, gender studies, history, and cultural studies – to bear on the archive, shedding light on memories, discourses, trauma, and activism.

Using a medical humanities framework, the editors explore the influence of historical representations of HIV/AIDS and stigma in a world where antiretroviral treatment has fundamentally altered the conditions under which many people diagnosed with HIV live. Organized into four sections, this book begins by introducing the archive and its role, setting it in a global context. The first part looks at methodological, legal, and ethical issues around archiving memories of the present, which are then used to construct histories of the past, something that can be particularly controversial when dealing with a socially stigmatized epidemic such as HIV/AIDS. The second section is devoted to analyses of particular films from the archive, looking at the portrayal of people living with HIV/AIDS, the narrative of HIV as a chronic illness, and the contemporary context of particular films. The third section looks at how stigma and trauma are negotiated in the material in the Face of AIDS film archive, discussing ideas about suffering and culpability. The final section contributes perspectives on and by the filmmaker as activist and auteur.

This interdisciplinary collection is placed at the intersection of medical humanities, sexuality studies and film and media studies, continuing a tradition of studies on the cultural and social understandings of HIV/AIDS.

Elisabet Björklund is a postdoctoral researcher at the Department of History of Science and Ideas at Uppsala University and Senior Lecturer in Film Studies at Linnaeus University, Sweden.

Mariah Larsson is Professor in Film Studies at Linnaeus University, Sweden.

Routledge Advances in the Medical Humanities

For more information about this series please visit
www.routledge.com/Routledge-Advances-in-Disability-Studies/book-series/RADS

A Visual History of HIV/AIDS

Exploring the Face of AIDS Film Archive

**Edited by Elisabet Björklund and
Mariah Larsson**

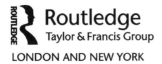

Routledge
Taylor & Francis Group

LONDON AND NEW YORK

First published 2019 by Routledge

2 Park Square, Milton Park, Abingdon, Oxfordshire OX14 4RN
52 Vanderbilt Avenue, New York, NY 10017

Routledge is an imprint of the Taylor & Francis Group, an informa business

First issued in paperback 2019

British Library Cataloguing-in-Publication Data
A catalogue record for this book is available from the British Library

Library of Congress Cataloging-in-Publication Data
Names: Bjørklund:, Elisabet, 1983- editor. | Larsson, Mariah, 1972- editor.
Title: A visual history of HIV/AIDS : exploring the face of AIDS film
archive / edited by Elisabet Björklund and Mariah Larsson.
Description: Abingdon, Oxon ; New York, NY : Routledge, 2018. |
Includes bibliographical references and index.
Identifiers: LCCN 2018010636| ISBN 9781138503243 (hardback) |
ISBN 9781315145310 (ebook)
Subjects: | MESH: Face of Aids (Organization) | HIV Infections |
Acquired Immunodeficiency Syndrome | Political Activism | Motion
Pictures | Archives | Sweden
Classification: LCC RA643.83 | NLM WC 503 | DDC
614.5/9939200222–dc23
LC record available at https://lccn.loc.gov/2018010636

ISBN: 978-1-138-50324-3 (hbk)
ISBN: 978-0-367-45749-5 (pbk)

Typeset in Times New Roman
by Wearset Ltd, Boldon, Tyne and Wear

Contents

Figures

Contributors

Marco Bacio is a double PhD student of sociology at the University of Milan, Italy (where he teaches sociology to undergraduate students), and of gender studies at Lund University, Sweden (where he teaches quantitative methods to postgraduate students). His research interests include LGBT studies, gender studies, sexualities, sex work, and sociology of culture. Since 2011, he is a research fellow at "GENDERS", the Centre for Gender and Equality in Research and Science, of the University of Milan.

Elisabet Björklund is a postdoctoral researcher at the Department of History of Science and Ideas at Uppsala University, Sweden, and senior lecturer in film studies at Linnaeus University, Sweden. She earned her PhD in 2013 with a dissertation on sex education films in Sweden and is co-editor (with Mariah Larsson) of *Swedish Cinema and the Sexual Revolution: Critical Essays* (2016).

Adam Brenthel is a researcher of art history and visual studies at the Department of Arts and Cultural Sciences, Lund University. Brenthel has a research interest in natural scientific scenarios of the future and defended his thesis on climate change, *The Drowning World*, in 2016. The analysis has proven applicable to challenges within the field of medical humanities. His most recent project researches the post-antibiotic era.

Dagmar Brunow is a senior lecturer in film studies at Linnaeus University, Sweden. She has published widely on questions of cultural memory and the archive, video, and the essay film, as well as feminist and queer filmmaking. Her current research project, "The Cultural Memory of Moving Images" (2016–2018), was financed by the Swedish Research Council. She is the author of *Remediating Transcultural Memory* (Berlin/Boston: de Gruyter, 2015).

Tommy Gustafsson holds a PhD in history and is Professor of film studies at Linnaeus University, Sweden. He has previously published *Masculinity in the Golden Age of Swedish Cinema: A Cultural Analysis of 1920s Films* (McFarland, 2014) and the anthology *Nordic Genre Film: Small Nation Film Cultures in the Global Marketplace* (with Pietari Kääpä, Edinburgh University Press, 2015).

Kristofer Hansson is a researcher and reader of ethnology at the Department of Arts and Cultural Sciences, Lund University. He did his PhD studies at Vård-alinstitutet, the Swedish Institute for Health Sciences. His research focus is cultural analysis of medical practice in health care and biomedical research. In recent years much of his research has related to citizen participation in new biomedical technologies.

Staffan Hildebrand is a journalist and filmmaker. He has worked for Swedish television and has made several fiction and documentary films, in particular with a focus on young people. Among them are *G – som i gemenskap* ("C – as in Community", 1983) and *Stockholmsnatt* ("Stockholm Night", 1987). For the past thirty years, he has been documenting the HIV/AIDS pandemic, resulting in the Face of AIDS film archive at Karolinska Institutet.

Martin Kristenson is a librarian at Karolinska Institutet University Library and project secretary of the Face of AIDS film archive.

Mariah Larsson is Professor of film studies at Linnaeus University, Sweden. Among her recent publications are *The Swedish Porn Scene: Exhibition Contexts, 8mm Pornography and the Sex Film* (Intellect, 2017), "Adapting Sex: Cultural Conceptions of Sexuality in Words and Images" in *Women of Ice and Fire* (Bloomsbury, 2016) and "The Death of Porn? An Autopsy of 'Scandinavian Sin' in the Twenty-first Century" in *A Companion to Nordic Cinema* (Wiley-Blackwell, 2016).

Desireé Ljungcrantz, PhD in gender studies from Linköping University, Sweden, wrote her dissertation on the cultural imaginaries and the experiences of living with HIV in a contemporary Swedish context. The thesis, *Skrubbsår. Berättelser om hur hiv erfars och föreställs i samtida Sverige* (2017), is published by Makadam. Desireé Ljungcrantz teaches and writes on normativities related to health, gender, sexuality, etc. within and outside academia.

Daniel Normark is a researcher at Uppsala Science and Technology Studies Centre, Uppsala University, and affiliated to the medical history and heritage unit, Karolinska Institutet. He holds a PhD in science and technology studies from the University of Gothenburg. Normark is currently working on the "masters of flavour", the introduction of sensory science in the twentieth century.

Fredrik B. Persson is a librarian at Karolinska Institutet University Library and the project manager of the Face of AIDS film archive.

Cirus Rinaldi, PhD, is a senior lecturer of the sociology of deviance at the Department of Culture and Society, University of Palermo, where he teaches genders, sexualities, and violence, LGBT studies, and queer theory. His main research topics are related to masculinity and violence, homophobia, deviance theory, and the sociology of sexualities. He is a member of the scientific committee of the Gender Studies section of AIS (the Italian Sociological Association).

Anna Sofia Rossholm is a senior lecturer in film studies at Linnaeus University. Her research focuses on the relation between film and other media. She has published numerous articles and book chapters in the fields of adaptation studies and screenwriting studies. Her latest book examines the process of screenwriting in Ingmar Bergman's filmmaking.

Beate Schirrmacher, PhD, is a senior lecturer in comparative literature at Linnaeus University and a member of the Linnaeus University Centre of Intermedial and Multimodal Studies. She received her PhD in 2012 from Stockholm University with a thesis on music in Günter Grass's prose. Her current research includes the relation of authenticity, witnessing and mediation.

David Thorsén is a senior lecturer at the Department of Education, Stockholm University. Thorsén's research and teaching interests include medical humanities, visual culture, media history, and the history of education. His previous research projects have explored the public and governmental responses to HIV and AIDS in Sweden in the 1980s and early 1990s, primarily the national information campaigns headed by the National Commission on AIDS ("AIDS-delegationen").

Paula A. Treichler holds a BA from Antioch College and a PhD in linguistics and psycholinguistics from the University of Rochester. Her book on the HIV/AIDS epidemic, *How to Have Theory in an Epidemic: Cultural Chronicles of AIDS* (Duke University Press, 1999), tracks the epidemic from the beginning; the book is widely cited in HIV scholarship and taught in university courses. She has been called a singularly important voice among the significant theorists on the AIDS crisis; her work has altered the field of cultural studies by establishing medicine as a legitimate object of investigation. She is presently completing *How to Use a Condom: Cultural History since 1853* (working title). She is Professor Emerita in Media and Cinema Studies at the University of Illinois at Urbana-Champaign.

Cecilia Trenter received her PhD in 1999 from the Department of History, Uppsala University, Sweden. She is a senior lecturer at Linnaeus University at the Department of Cultural Studies. Her research focuses on the field of social memory. Trenter has been working with representations of the past in fiction and heritage adaptations, for example in her ongoing research on adaptations of memorials into fictional historical drama in films.

Preface

Faces, meanings, archives

Paula A. Treichler

It is my privilege to introduce this collection of essays about the Face of AIDS film archive cataloged and housed in Karolinska Institutet in Stockholm, Sweden. When Stockholm was chosen as the site for the 1988 Fourth International AIDS Conference, the Institute, as the leading Swedish medical university, was a logical host and organizer. Already familiar with the work of Swedish filmmaker Staffan Hildebrand, notably his short documentary *AIDS: Perceptions about a Reality*, the Institute's president, Dr. Hans Wigzell, commissioned Hildebrand to create a film to open the conference. The goal was to emphasize the global realities and multiple individuals and communities affected by the epidemic, and to make a film that was arresting, adventurous, and compassionate. The result was the 1988 *Crossover: The Global Impact of AIDS*. Its success at the conference led the Institute to propose to Hildebrand a remarkable follow-up project: to document the epidemic on film *for the next thirty years*. Accordingly, Hildebrand worked on the project from 1987 to 2017. The Face of AIDS film archive is the realization of that project.

Although Sweden may not be the first country you would associate with HIV/AIDS, several compelling reasons argue for its importance. Sweden is the first country to have achieved the UNAIDS/WHO Treatment for All goal for HIV by 2020.[1] Its commitment to the film archive is in keeping with the country's early engagement with HIV/AIDS, initiating a proactive program superior to that of many other nations. Karolinska Institutet was well-equipped to oversee, host, and organize the 1988 International AIDS Conference. In a significant departure from past conferences – two of the previous three had been held in the U.S. – the Stockholm organizers insisted on the global nature of the epidemic including its growing presence in sub-Saharan Africa. Karolinska Institutet participates in awarding the Nobel Prize for Physiology or Medicine and in 2008, twenty years after the Stockholm conference, the selection committee awarded the prize jointly to French scientists Luc Montagnier and Françoise Barré-Sinousi of the Pasteur Institute in Paris for their significant biomedical work on identifying HIV, the "AIDS virus." Beyond Sweden's biomedical credentials, the country's social welfare governance structure tends to foster projects and initiatives aimed at the public good. Within that overarching ethos, Sweden offers, too, a long tradition of production of and respect for cinema as an art and industry along with an established international reputation for quality and prestige. Finally, Sweden is home to the legendary scientist Carl Linnaeus, whose taxonomies revolutionized recognition, classification, and categorization of the natural world. Still in use today around the world, Linnaeus's system is part of a long Swedish archival tradition – some say "the best in the world."

It is fitting that Linnaeus University is home to the editors of this collection on the Face of AIDS film archive. Faculty members in the Department of Film and Literature Mariah Larsson and Elisabet Björklund are accomplished teachers and scholars whose work demonstrates brainy analyses of Swedish film history and specialized cinematic genres. They recognized early on the unique significance of the Face of AIDS film archive as a resource for the study of the AIDS epidemic; as a body of work relevant to practitioners in many scholarly disciplines and interest areas; and as a film collection with its own intrinsic cinematic interest. Contributors to this volume representing several academic and professional fields demonstrate various approaches to and perspectives on the archive. But their approaches are by no means exhaustive: the archive is massive, rich in diverse material, and user-friendly. It is hoped that this book is the first in what will be a series of publications about the archive.

* * *

When I first engaged with Staffan Hildebrand's archival project, its title concerned me. Throughout the epidemic, "The Face of AIDS" has been a recurring and reliable media trope, even a media cliché, to signal how some decision-maker chooses to represent "AIDS." The selected "face" rarely correlates with number of cases, new epidemiological data, or new information about transmission and spread. Rather, each face communicates in shorthand a particular narrative about HIV/AIDS at a particular time.[2] Each face projects a frozen moment in which *this* face is a key to understanding the whole epidemic, or evaluating its dangers, or alerting the public to some new AIDS threat – or, it must be acknowledged, selling media products. With few exceptions, the narrative structure behind each portrait suggests that the face (1) exemplifies a known "risk group," (2) identifies a seemingly new "risk group," (3) shows us the face of the Other, or (4) reveals that the epidemic is not what we think it is.

Consider the famous *Newsweek* cover story of August 1985 which informed the public at large that Rock Hudson had AIDS and was traveling to Paris for treatment. Though an open secret in Hollywood, the news that a leading movie star celebrated for his masculinity was gay was a shocking lesson to the general public (though a lesson not universally grasped: "If Rock Hudson can get it," remarked one man, "nobody's safe!"). But, as the first top celebrity to reveal that he had AIDS, he was a media magnet. There was some grousing in gay publications that it took a famous gay man to get the epidemic on the radar, yet, according to longitudinal media studies, Rock Hudson's illness and death constituted a critical turning point in the evolution of consciousness about AIDS: it significantly increased the average number of AIDS stories per month and expanded newspaper coverage almost threefold.[3] The quantity of coverage subsequently subsided, but, as would be true for subsequent "celebrity AIDS" cases, it never returned to its earlier level. As the Face of AIDS, the image of Hudson gaunt, frail, and shockingly changed was frozen in time, and has served as an iconic image ever since.

The Face of AIDS film archive is most definitely about *faces* of AIDS, in the plural. *Crossover*, the film that opened the 1988 conference, makes clear that the film, like the archive as a whole, captures the project's goal of showing a diversity of people, countries, and cultures infected and affected by the epidemic. In the prelude, voices that we will hear again later in the film attribute different meanings to the epidemic: an Australian judge cites the creation of "otherness" as a driver of the epidemic; a black rapper is sampled; a New York cabbie says that "by the time there's a cure, half of America will be dead"; a white man in a hospital bed presents himself as what happens "if you fuck around"; a twenty-something kid in Australia tells Hildebrand, "Look at us now – what do we live in? Bombs, AIDS, you name it, you know. I'm not proud of the world today that the grownups have given us"; a sick Australian man with Kaposi's reflects on the body as spiritual as well as physical; an American white kid in his twenties says "AIDS, man? AIDS. The only way you can get AIDS is if you're a homo"; a little girl says "AIDS is death"; and a scientist calls AIDS "a time bomb for the entire world." *Crossover* thus portrays the epidemic's global reach through countries, communities, and individuals. Unlike many documentaries on HIV/AIDS, *Crossover* does not explicitly offer didactic "lessons"; rather, the film speaks through the voices of its subjects. The archive's title, "The Face of AIDS," emphasizes, too, that the human, social, and indeed corporeal dimensions of the epidemic are as important to understand as the strictly scientific and biomedical. Interestingly, many of Hildebrand's interviews with scientists and clinicians show their human faces as they speak in very personal terms about their engagement with the epidemic.[4] The archive also makes accessible *changing* faces of AIDS over time (from 1987 to 2017) and place (Hildebrand filmed on every continent except Antarctica).

As I sampled the archive and read Hildebrand's commentaries, I was struck not only by the breadth of the project but by the filmmaker's continuing energy, curiosity, and goodwill as he encountered many kinds of people, projects, and venues. In Uganda, for example, trucks crossing the rural countryside had long served as images (if not precisely faces) of AIDS; having sexual encounters along their routes, the drivers were indicted as the carriers of AIDS to nonurban areas. Staffan Hildebrand is the only journalist I know who actually talked to them directly: "Did you have sex with anyone last night?" The truck drivers, like so many others, are faces that become part of the Face of AIDS film archive. Hildebrand is now, as thirty years of filmmaking come to an end, returning to some of the earlier people and places he filmed to explore their responses to their earlier appearances and to hear their reports of changes in the epidemic. As he connects and reconnects with AIDS hotspots, irresistible people, innovative events, and officially important scientific and medical meetings, Hildebrand creates an archive that is never singular, faces of AIDS that are never archetypes.

* * *

But I would like to return to "The Face of AIDS" as a recurrent media label. In contrast to the diversity and plurality of faces in the Face of AIDS film archive, even the few examples I cite here indicate that the words "The Face of AIDS" are neither bland nor neutral but rather constitute a singular name with its own history and power of signification. Its use typically consists of a single face, perhaps a single figure (rarely a gallery of faces): in each case the image stands in for an unknown number of infected Others, all too often denoting guilt or innocence. The precise title "Face of AIDS" may explicitly label the image, or be mentioned in the text, or simply be implied. The face suggests, confirms, or challenges what the public (reader/viewer/audience) thinks it already knows. In the first decade of the epidemic, the "Face of AIDS" was usually assumed to be a gay white man, the leading member of the original "4-H club" (homosexuals, hemophiliacs, heroin users, Haitians).[5] Because the mainstream media had yet to find ways of representing homosexuals, gay men at first appeared in distant shots of Castro Street in San Francisco or as gaunt dying figures, always alone, waiting to die. Photographer Nicholas Nixon's *People with AIDS* set the gold standard for this genre: those pictured in his book are wraiths, their arms all bones, their ribs like victims of starvation. In such photos, AIDS is a death sentence, but their suffering is rendered elegiac and in some sense universal. Infected intravenous users of illegal drugs were characterized in images and texts in equally predictable ways by the media: huddled in dark alleys or dirty crack houses or dying in hospital beds hooked up to very different drugs. A notorious example is the 1988 *Frontline* documentary about Fabian Bridges, a poor, black IV drug user and sex worker filmed as he sought money, drugs, and sex in the streets of Houston. As Douglas Crimp has written, every epidemic produces, indeed requires, a Typhoid Mary. First it was Gaetan Dugas, the French Canadian airline steward who was early targeted as AIDS's Patient Zero. Here it is Fabian, shocking PBS viewers (as well as the filmmakers) with what they saw as his promiscuous sexual encounters knowing he was infected.[6]

Rock Hudson, Gaetan Dugas, Fabian Bridges, and Nixon's skeletal portraits made visible and reaffirmed what the public at this point believed it knew about AIDS and the unfortunate souls most likely to get it and die. So the July 1985 cover of *Life* magazine was a shock. The "Face of AIDS" cover story presented unfamiliar faces to the public, appearing to contradict conventional wisdom and threaten the official assurances that "the general public is not at risk." In living color, photos of three people with AIDS looked out at readers: an African American soldier in uniform, saluting; an attractive young white woman, looking desolate; and Patrick Burk, with his white all-American nuclear family (mom, dad, daughter, son). In bold red letters, the cover warned "now no one is safe from AIDS." The pictures and headline together were clearly designed as a wake-up call and to affirm, perhaps, the prevailing medical and media mantra that "AIDS is an equal opportunity disease." Certainly, these faces of AIDS looked different from those mentioned above. But in fact those pictured represented known "risk groups": the soldier was the recipient of a contaminated blood transfusion, the young woman had slept with a bisexual man, and Patrick Burk was a man with hemophilia whose wife was also infected. This enabled *Life* to conclude that "AIDS remains within the original risk groups" and "the general public is safe." Wake-up calls are all to the good, but bait and switch calls are not helpful.

* * *

I intend these examples to be illustrative, not comprehensive. Many more come to mind: Ryan White, Princess Diana shaking hands with "an AIDS victim," Kimberly Bergalis, Freddy Mercury, and of course Magic Johnson. Except for Bergalis, these others ultimately had some positive interpretations and consequences. In the Ryan White case, the face of AIDS was that of an HIV+ schoolboy reviled by his Indiana community and school. Another community welcomed him and his family and he soon became a heroic figure – one who refused to use his youth and innocence to separate himself from people with AIDS typically deemed "guilty." Elton John played at his funeral, but, more remarkably, his case led to the creation of the Ryan White Act, which continues to provide comprehensive health care for people with HIV and AIDS (see Dawson and Kates 2015).

Among these early images, these frozen symbols of AIDS, are photos from countries whose citizens have little opportunity to speak for themselves. Today, the situation is different, with far more egalitarian circulation of images and information worldwide. But when Haitians were first identified with AIDS, their pictures took the predictable form of "Third World images," as we in "the First World" might expect them to look. A highly visible 1987 story for *Life* by physician-author Richard Selzer, for example, is titled "A Mask on the Face of Death." Striking photographs of gaunt, exhausted patients in squalid hospital corridors testify to the truth the article will claim. In a narrative that will become familiar, officials deny the presence of AIDS on the island while "the view from the street" adds a conspiracy trope to the official line: "AIDS!" says a prostitute Selzer interviews. "There is no such thing. It is a false disease invented by the American government to take advantage of the poor countries" (Treichler 1999: 102–103).[7] She is photographed on a bed wearing red (as sex workers often are in AIDS stories). The "Mask" evokes denial of AIDS's existence as well as conventional assumptions that Haiti is culturally exotic: we are to take for granted that Selzer, the trained American physician, can see through the mask. The "Mask on the Face of Death" asserts, finally, that AIDS is a death sentence.[8] As I recount in my book on the AIDS epidemic, another "third world" photograph, this one from sub-Saharan Africa, demonstrates the ease with which images can travel, leaving their captions and contexts behind. Taken by Ed Hooper, the photo shows an emaciated woman "in native garb" framed in the doorway of her home, holding a small, thin baby on her lap. Reprinted in numerous publications, the photo is given various captions: "Ugandan AIDS victims," "Two victims: Ugandan barmaid and son," and the like; in one story, the photo is used to illustrate the explosion of AIDS in sub-Saharan Africa, in another, to claim that the epidemic in Africa has been greatly exaggerated. In his 1990 memoir *Slim*, Ed Hooper, working and living for years as a photographer in Uganda, knew the woman and her son. He expresses discomfort with the ways the photo was taken up without context. His own caption reads "Florence and Ssengabi, sitting outside their hut in Gwanda. Florence died one month after this photograph was taken; her son died four months later."[9]

A very different transformation of meaning, this time from the American heartland, took place around Therese Frare's photograph, published in *Life* in November 1990 and hailed as "the photo that changed the Face of AIDS" (Cosgrove 2014). In a series of pictures, Frare told the story of David Kirby, a gay activist in San Francisco in the late 1980s; when he learned he was HIV+ and grew ill, he asked his family in his small Ohio town – from whom, like many others in his situation, he was estranged – if he could come home to die. They welcomed him, and Frare was given permission by him and his family to chronicle this experience. The famous photo shows Kirby close to death, surrounded by his family, in a moving tableau so iconic that United Colors of Benetton used it for a controversial ad that enhanced the photo's drama, in part by alluding to such death scenes in high art. The photo and its memorializing by Benetton were controversial because of a continuing conflict over the meaning of AIDS. Is an AIDS death the tragic yet inevitable and natural outcome of a horrifying event in human history – like plague, the Spanish flu epidemic, cholera? The Frare photograph, enhanced by the Benetton rendering, embodies this humanistic frame that sees death as tragic yet redeemed and transcended by art and compassion. Challenging this view were those who refused to accept such high-minded yet passive fatalism and instead saw AIDS deaths as calls to action and intervention: Certainly AIDS was terrible and often fatal but *not inevitable* – rather, its continued fatalities and spread were enabled by repressive legislation, homophobia, and government failure to fund education, intervention, and treatment research.[10] I would argue that this orchestration of new meanings by activists like Larry Kramer and activist groups like Gay Men's Health Crisis and ACT UP amounted to a redefinition of the epidemic that in turn brought about widespread changes in policies and practices.[11]

Conclusion

The title "The Face of AIDS" as employed for the Face of AIDS film archive is a legitimate synecdoche for all persons infected with and affected by HIV/AIDS and captures the encompassing and inclusive intent of the film archive project. But tension remains between that reasonable and easily recognizable archive title and, as I have argued here, "The Face of AIDS" as a site that throughout the epidemic has represented contested meanings, conflicting agendas, special interests, alternative perspectives, and changing understandings of HIV/AIDS. While seemingly straightforward, a given "Face of AIDS" may be welcomed, another resisted or reviled. Over the course of the epidemic, the term has done duty for many groups and agendas, in some cases resulting in important policy choices with clear material consequences.

The value of the Face of AIDS film archive is that it refuses to designate any face as *the* face of AIDS: with its plurality, eclecticism, and sweep of people, times, and places, the archive thus performs a crucial corrective function. In Hildebrand's collection, photo images are not frozen in time and meanings and lessons are not forced upon the viewer. The scholars and professionals represented in this book select faces and draw meanings according to their various investigations. The contrast between these two distinct uses of "The Face of AIDS" illustrates different approaches to representation, at the same time offering guidance in the reading of media images that goes beyond the HIV/AIDS epidemic. Responding to an image requires more than a cognitive, emotional, or political response. Whether it is "the Face of Washington," "Face of Polio," "Face of Climate Change," or "Face of AIDS," the image requires attention to framing, to visual and narrative genres, to sources, to allusions to existing images, to the intent and credentials of the producer and disseminator of the image, to context, and to consequences.

Notes

1 Treatment for All seeks to end the global HIV/AIDS epidemic by 2030. To do so, the interim goal is that by 2020 90 percent of people with HIV worldwide should know their diagnosis, 90 percent of people diagnosed should be on antiretroviral therapy, and 90 percent of those on ART should be virally suppressed.
2 See reports and bulletins from the Kaiser Family Foundation on longitudinal media coverage as well as other health issues (kff.org; see also Shilts 1987). It is important to keep in mind that for the first 15–20 years of the epidemic there was no Internet, no World Wide Web, no social media.
3 For more on media coverage, including global coverage, see Treichler 1999; Treichler *et al.* 1998; and Mann and Tarantola 1996. This last book is perhaps the first book to provide a comprehensive and complex overview of the global epidemic. Despite its date, it remains an indispensable resource. Hildebrand's interview with Mann is in the Face of AIDS film archive.
4 Gripping oral histories of U.S. physicians' experiences with the epidemic are collected in Bayer and Oppenheimer (2000) and of the South African epidemic in Oppenheimer and Bayer (2007).
5 As shorthand, the "4-H club" was never used scientifically but, however bogus, it entered into wide usage in journalistic accounts, though often used ironically. "Hookers" was originally the fourth "H" until female prostitutes in the U.S. had unexpectedly few symptoms so Haitians got the honor.
6 These portrayals were lauded as artistic and informative. They were also sharply criticized by such cultural critics and AIDS activists as Douglas Crimp (1992), John Greyson (1987; 1993), and Bordowitz and Carlomusto (1989). See also Gould (2009) and Patton (1990).
7 As I've often argued, "conspiracy theories" should not be dismissed out of hand as ignorant, dangerous, or crazy. Though they may be seen as misguided in terms of

science and facts, they nevertheless provide useful information from the ground (i.e., people's lived experience), suggest how scientific and public health materials might better speak to people's existing understandings, and offer possibilities for effective collaboration with local knowledge.

8 Structural violence affecting women in Haiti is explored by Farmer *et al.* (1996).

9 Analyses of the struggles surrounding women and AIDS in sub-Saharan Africa include Booth (2004) and Susser (2009). Randolph (2017) details the appearance of Rae Lewis-Thornton on the cover of the African American magazine *Ebony*. A well-dressed, well-educated professional African American woman, Lewis-Thornton's challenge of prevailing stereotypes had considerable impact on women of color, especially young women.

10 John James, who founded and edited the weekly newsletter *AIDS Treatment News* from nearly the beginning of the epidemic, has written that this quest for "the beautiful death" was a significant barrier to serious discussion of treatment possibilities.

11 In Treichler (1999) I explore the conversion of meanings to definitions in relation to the AIDS epidemic. A more systematic analysis, that of dissent and controversy among AIDS scientists, can be found in Fujimura and Chou (1994).

Bibliography

Bayer, Ronald and G. Oppenheimer (2000). *AIDS Doctors: Voices from the Epidemic.* Oxford: Oxford University Press.

Björklund, Elisabet and Mariah Larsson (2016). "Introduction: Beyond Swedish Summers," in Elisabet Bjorklund and Mariah Larsson (eds), *Swedish Cinema and the Sexual Revolution: Critical Essays.* Jefferson, NC: McFarland.

Björklund, Elisabet and Mariah Larsson, eds (2016). *Swedish Cinema and the Sexual Revolution: Critical Essays.* Jefferson, NC: McFarland.

Booth, Karen (2004). *Local Women, Global Science: Fighting AIDS in Kenya.* Bloomington, IN: Indiana University Press.

Bordowitz, Gregg and Jean Carlomusto (1989). "Seize Control of the FDA," Living with AIDS series. New York: Gay Men's Health Crisis. Video.

Cosgrove, Ben (2014). "The Photo That Changed the Face of AIDS," *Time*, November 25.

Crimp, Douglas, ed. (1988). *AIDS: Cultural Analysis/Cultural Activism.* Cambridge, MA: MIT Press.

Crimp, Douglas (1992). "Portraits of People with AIDS," in Lawrence Grossberg, Cary Nelson, and Paula A Treichler (eds), *Cultural Studies.* New York: Routledge.

Dawson, Lindsey and Jennifer Kates (2015). *The Ryan White Program and Insurance Purchasing in the ACA Era: An Early Look at Five States.* Menlo Park CA: Kaiser Family Foundation, April 14. www.kff.org.

Farmer, Paul, Margaret Connors, and Janie Simmons, eds (1996). *Women, Poverty, and AIDS: Sex, Drugs, and Structural Violence.* Monroe, ME: Common Courage.

Fujimura, Joan and Danny Chou (1994). "Dissent in Science: Styles of Scientific Practice and the Controversy over the Cause of AIDS," *Social Science and Medicine* 38(8): 1017–1036.

Gould, Deborah B. (2009). *Moving Politics: Emotion and ACT UP's Fight against AIDS.* Chicago, IL, and London: University of Chicago Press.

Greyson, John, director (1987). *The ADS Epidemic.* Toronto: V Tape (available online).

Greyson, John, director (1993). *Zero Patience.* Toronto: Zero Patience Productions. Film (available on DVD and online).

Hooper, Ed (1990). *Slim: A Reporter's Own Story of AIDS in East Africa*. London: Bodley Head.

James, John S., ed. (1991). *AIDS Treatment News*. Newsletter published April 1986–December 1993. Collected in three volumes.

Kaiser Family Foundation (1996). *AIDS Media Study: 1981–1994*. Menlo Park CA: Kaiser Family Foundation. See also the many follow-up studies by Kaiser at kff.org.

Larsson, Mariah (2017). *The Swedish Porn Scene: Exhibition Contexts, 8mm Pornography, and the Sex Film*. Bristol and Chicago, IL: Intellect.

Oppenheimer, G. and Ronald Bayer (2007). *Shattered Dreams?: An Oral History of the South African AIDS Epidemic*. Oxford: Oxford University Press.

Patton, Cindy (1990). *Inventing AIDS*. New York: Routledge.

Randolph, Carolyn A. (2017). *Black Women, HIV/AIDS, and the Media: Communicating an Epidemic in the Hip Hop Era*. Unpublished doctoral dissertation, University of Illinois at Urbana-Champaign. See especially Chapter 4: "'Diva Living with Aids': Rae Lewis-Thornton and the Crafting of a Public Persona."

Shilts, Randy (1987). *And the Band Played On: People, Politics, and the AIDS Epidemic*. New York: St. Martin's.

Susser, Ida (2009). *AIDS, Sex, and Culture: Global Politics and Survival in South Africa*. Hoboke, NJ: Wiley-Blackwell.

Tomes, Nancy (2007). "Celebrity Disease," in Leslie J. Reagan, Nancy Tomes, and Paula A. Treichler (eds), *Medicine's Moving Pictures: Medicine, Health, and Bodies in American Film and Television*. Rochester, NY: University of Rochester Press.

Treichler, Paula A (1999). *How to Have Theory in an Epidemic: Cultural Chronicles of AIDS*. Durham, NY: Duke University Press.

Treichler, Paula A., Daniel E. McGee, Maria V. Ruiz, and Niranjan Karnik (1998). "The Legacy of AIDS: Global Media Coverage of Emerging Infectious Diseases," poster presentation, Twelfth International Conference on AIDS, Geneva, July 1.

Acknowledgments

First of all, we would like to thank the contributors, who brought the perspectives of their different disciplines and research areas to the Face of AIDS film archive and made the collection what it is. Moreover, Linnaeus University has supported us in the organizing of workshops and the editing of this volume.

The Face of AIDS film archive consists of material filmed by Staffan Hildebrand and then indexed and archived by Karolinska Institutet's University Library. The original idea to document the HIV/AIDS pandemic on film, however, came from Hans Wigzell at Karolinska Institutet. Martin Kristenson and Fredrik B. Persson have done a wonderful job organizing the archive and making it searchable. In addition, they have been very helpful with the illustrations of this book.

In June 2017, editors and contributors convened for a workshop at Linnaeus University for discussion of the work in progress. At this workshop, Paula A. Treichler was an invited respondent and commented on all present contributors' chapter drafts. Her input was absolutely essential and it was a privilege to have such a knowledgeable and insightful scholar provide feedback.

We would also like to thank Sara Johnsdotter at Malmö University for helpful comments and advice during our work.

An ethical vetting application for this project was approved on September 19, 2017.

Finally, and as always, our warmest love and gratitude go to our families: Lasse, Naima, and Arvid, and Olle, Albert, Martha, and Kinsey the boxer dog.

Introduction

Elisabet Björklund and Mariah Larsson

The Face of AIDS film archive at Karolinska Institutet consists of approximately 700 hours of unedited and edited footage, shot over a period of thirty years and all over the world by Swedish filmmaker and journalist Staffan Hildebrand. The material documents the HIV/AIDS pandemic and includes scenes from conferences and rallies, and interviews with activists, physicians, people living with HIV, and researchers. Since it is also a documentation over time, it represents a global historical development from the early years of the AIDS crisis to a situation in which it is possible to live a normal life with the HIV virus (at least in the Western world) (http://kib.ki.se/en/faceofaids). Most of the footage is shot in North America (35 percent) and Europe (22 percent), but the archive also contains footage from Africa (21 percent), Asia (16 percent), South America (4 percent), and Australia (2 percent). *A Visual History of HIV/AIDS* explores the archive by bringing scholars from different academic disciplines together. It also brings in the voice of the filmmaker, looking back at his work, while the contributing scholars – from media and film studies, medical history, gender studies, history, and cultural studies – deliver a multidisciplinary spectrum of analyses.

The HIV/AIDS pandemic has been formative for a large share of the twentieth and early twenty-first centuries. Beginning in the early 1980s as an epidemic that appeared to concern only men who had sex with men, it started by being constructed as a "gay disease" in a discourse shaped by sexual moralism and homophobia that seemingly irrevocably attached a strong and shameful stigma to AIDS. It continued as a "moral panic" or social scare when it became apparent that also the heterosexual community could receive, transmit, and carry the virus, only to be later transferred to be regarded as a symptom and a peril of the "dark continent," Africa, and as a result of the global injustices in the unequal power and economic balance of the world. When antiretroviral treatment became available in the mid-1990s, the reality of HIV and AIDS changed, and today the most immediate threat to humankind seems to have passed.[1] The number of both HIV transmissions and AIDS-related deaths in the world are declining (UNAIDS 2017: 4–7). Although no vaccine or cure has been found, antiretroviral treatment is a medical success story, providing people living with HIV the opportunity to live a next-to-normal life. Both preexposure prophylaxis and postexposure prophylaxis are in existence and accessible in some parts of the world. From a very optimistic perspective, one could claim that HIV and AIDS have lost their immediate urgency as a major threat to humankind and that, thereby, the "epidemic of signification" that Paula A. Treichler once described AIDS as, has petered out (Treichler 1999).

Accordingly, one could pose the question: Why an edited collection on HIV and AIDS now? And why, in particular, one that approaches the subject from, mainly, a humanities perspective? One could even argue that the work that remains lies in the realm of prevention and education, access to medical care in the form of HIV testing and antiretroviral treatment, and vigilance from the bio-medical community.

However, at this point in time, people are still alive who remember the early days of the epidemic. There are still people living who were on the verge of death in 1996, when antiretroviral treatment became available and saved their lives. The AIDS epidemic began, roughly, a generation ago, and, since the immediate concern of a pandemic threatening humankind has passed, now comes a time for retrospection. In her book *Representations of HIV and AIDS – Visibility Blue/s*, from 2000, Gabriele Griffin discussed how HIV and AIDS had then gone from being visible almost everywhere in Western media of the late 1980s and early 1990s to being almost invisible around the turn of the century (Griffin 2000). Nevertheless, in recent years, there have appeared a great number of films, books, and TV series that tell the history of HIV and AIDS, and suggest that the epidemic is now gaining a new visibility. Examples include the American miniseries *Angels in America* (Mike Nichols, 2003), the documentaries *We Were Here* (David Weissman and Bill Weber, 2011), *How to Survive a Plague* (David France, 2012; expanded into a book in 2016), and *Desert Migration* (Daniel F. Cardone, 2015), and the fiction films *Dallas Buyers Club* (Jean-Marc Vallée, 2013) and the French *120 BPM* (Robin Campillo, 2017). In Sweden, comedian and author Jonas Gardell published the trilogy *Torka aldrig tårar utan handskar* (*Don't Ever Wipe Tears without Gloves*) in 2012–2013, mixing fiction and documentary, about AIDS among young gay men in Stockholm in the 1980s. The three books were made into a miniseries in 2012 directed by Simon Kaijser. The 1995 Australian memoir *Holding the Man* by Timothy Conigrave was made into a stage play in 2006 (directed by Tommy Murphy) and adapted into a film in 2015 (directed by Neil Armfield).

The list could go on, but still it indicates a general perception that we need to look back – in order to remember, to understand, to make the past coherent, to draw conclusions that were not possible to make when the present called for all attention. In one of the documentaries in the Face of AIDS film archive, *The Longest Journey Is the Journey Within* (Staffan Hildebrand, 2015), the prot-agonist at one point observes that "all the cruelty and meaninglessness get some kind of significance when what happened becomes a narrative." Moreover, the number of films and TV series produced suggests that audiovisual representa-tions are at the core of this retrospection, either with footage in documentaries as a visible evidence of the past or as the reconstruction of bygone days in drama and fiction. For this edited collection, the Face of AIDS film archive has offered a unique documentation of the HIV/AIDS pandemic, as historical source documents and as narratives and fragments of memories, experiences, trauma, and activism during a period of over thirty years. By studying the material in the archive, one purpose of the volume is to contribute to a retrospective understanding of the pandemic and its significations.

Furthermore, the HIV diagnosis still carries a stigma and awakens fear in the general public. In a Swedish study published in 2017, one third of the respondents would not perform first aid on a person if they knew that he or she was living with HIV (Noaks ark 2017). What seems to be important is that we do not stop talking about HIV and AIDS. Although, perhaps, silence does not necessarily equal death anymore – as famously stated in the logo of U.S. AIDS activist group ACT UP (see e.g., Griffin 2000: 36–38) – silence will undermine some of the progress that has been made as well as reproduce the stigma of HIV. A second purpose is thus to continue the discussion and critical analysis of HIV/AIDS in order to create awareness of the processes that have shaped cultural understandings of the epidemic, which are still persisting, and to address how contemporary representations relate to historical ones.

A third purpose of this volume is to demonstrate the usefulness of the Face of AIDS film archive. We are, in a sense, exploring the archive's potential. One could say that we, within the necessary ethical parameters, set our contributors loose in the archive to see what they could find and what they could do. This is also the reason why we have invited scholars from different backgrounds to contribute to the volume. It has been our aim to create a multidisciplinary book that demonstrates how the material in the Face of AIDS film archive may be studied from various perspectives. The result is a collection that represents many different approaches to the material, which will, hopefully, stimulate future work on the archive.

This brings us to yet another question: why a Swedish archive documenting the HIV/AIDS pandemic? Sweden was somewhat peripheral to the pandemic, and although the Fourth International AIDS Conference – when Hildebrand's project of documenting HIV/AIDS commenced – was held in Stockholm, and several Swedish researchers were important in the struggle against HIV and AIDS, Sweden does not, in general, seem very central to the international efforts of ending AIDS. Nevertheless, Sweden comes across as a both paradoxical and logical starting point for an archive of HIV and AIDS. There is a twentieth-century history of being liberal in relation to sexuality as well as a strong tradition of sexual education for children and young people, beginning in the mid-1950s (e.g., Lennerhed 1994; Björklund 2012). At the same time, there is also a tradition of repressive measures in relation to public health that was manifested very clearly during the years of "AIDS scare" in the late 1980s (cf. Henriksson and Ytterberg 1992). For instance, HIV/AIDS was placed under the Contagious Disease Act in 1985 (Bredström 2008: 59–61), among other things obliging people living with HIV, under the penalty of law, to inform potential partners prior to sexual contact about their HIV status. In 1987, gay saunas and other similar meeting places where men might have sex with other men were

4 Elisabet Björklund and Mariah Larsson

forced to close because of the "sauna law" (Henriksson 1988; 1995; Bredström 2008: 68).

During the same period, Sweden self-consciously took on the role of world conscience, acting out as a successful welfare state on moral high ground. In development aid, Sweden has been a generous donor, extending the practice of the welfare state to developing countries (Engh 2009). Hildebrand's project has, through the years, been partly funded by both the Ministry for Foreign Affairs and the Swedish foreign aid organization SIDA (Swedish International Development Cooperation Agency), thus suggesting a relationship between his documentation of the HIV/AIDS epidemic and Swedish foreign affairs and foreign aid. In addition, according to Engh (2009), Sweden's development aid has to a large extent focused on issues of reproduction. To this can be added what is today most often referred to as SRHR, sexual and reproductive health and rights, which the RFSU (the Swedish Association for Sexuality Education) has been increasingly involved with since the 1990s (www.rfsu.se/sv/Internationellt/Bakgrund-och-historik).

Accordingly, against this backdrop, it may not be surprising that a Swedish institution (Karolinska Institutet) suggested the project and that a Swedish journalist and filmmaker took it upon himself to realize it. However, although the film archive originated in Sweden and is housed in Sweden, the material in the archive is global. In itself, the archive is therefore not only, or even mostly, pertaining to issues relevant to Sweden, as many of the chapters in this volume illustrate. The global scope of the Face of AIDS film archive is one of its most significant qualities.

Background/previous research

During the 1980s and 1990s, AIDS activists and scholars within the humanities and social sciences started to give attention to the representation and social construction of the epidemic, and to how it was handled in Western media. Some of the most influential contributions include Simon Watney's *Policing Desire: Pornography, AIDS, and the Media* (1987), Susan Sontag's *AIDS and Its Metaphors* (1990 [1988]), Cindy Patton's *Inventing AIDS* (1990), and Paula A. Treichler's *How To Have Theory in an Epidemic: Cultural Chronicles of AIDS* (1999). Our project continues in this tradition of "critical HIV/AIDS researchers," described by Anna Bredström in her study of ethnicity and Swedish HIV/AIDS policy as a body of scholarly work that from a variety of theoretical perspectives interrogates the meaning and discourses of HIV/AIDS, often in some sort of agreement with or inspired by AIDS activism (Bredström 2008: 26). As a study of a film archive, the volume also connects to studies of HIV and AIDS in audiovisual media. There have been many studies made with this focus, especially from a North American perspective, examining mainstream Hollywood fiction films (e.g., McKinnon 1992; Hart 2000) and alternative productions (Juhasz 1995; Hallas 2009), as well as educational films (Eberwein 1999: 162–172; Milliken 2003: 315–380). Through focusing on a film archive, the volume thus adds new perspectives to already existing ones. As such, the study also contributes to the growing field of archival film studies, which has become an increasingly relevant area of research in the digital age (see e.g., Snickars and Vonderau 2009; Brunow 2017).

Much knowledge about the sociocultural significations of HIV/AIDS originates from and deals with the Anglo-American area. By bringing attention to the Face of AIDS film archive, we wish to accomplish a shift in focus and in historiography, which will contribute to a more multifaceted understanding of the meanings and discourses of HIV/AIDS. This is a relevant change of vantage point, as HIV/AIDS never was simply a "gay disease," an "American problem," a "Sub-Saharan disaster" or a "third world menace," a "stigma," or "moral panic," although it has been all of these things as well. The volume thus also contributes to the Swedish history of HIV and AIDS. A number of studies have been carried out which explore HIV and AIDS in a Swedish context and the Swedish HIV/AIDS policy from different perspectives (e.g., Ljung 2001; Bredström 2008; Thorsén 2013), but studies looking at Swedish audiovisual representations of the epidemic are sparse.

The volume is also a contribution to the growing field of medical humanities, the objective of which is to study the connection between human cultural life and medicine and vice versa. By providing multidisciplinary humanities perspectives on a medical phenomenon and by using various methods to frame and analyze filmed material, our aim is to broaden the ways of approaching and understanding a medical history. The volume thus connects to studies on moving images and medicine, for example Lisa Cartwright's *Screening the Body: Tracing Medicine's Visual Culture* (1995), Kirsten Ostherr's *Medical Visions: Producing the Patient through Film, Television, and Imaging Technologies* (2013), and edited volumes like *Cultural Sutures: Medicine and Media* (Friedman 2004) and *Medicine's Moving Pictures* (Reagan, Tomes, and Treichler 2008).

HIV and AIDS in hindsight: terminology, problems, and advantages

As anyone who works with HIV and AIDS in any way soon realizes, this is an area where vocabulary is of outmost importance, not least because of the stigma attached to the diagnosis of HIV but also, and related to that stigma, the epidemic has struck most strongly people who are, in one way or another, oppressed, marginalized, disenfranchised, or poor: the gay community, people with hemophilia, people who inject drugs, sex workers, migrants, people who have been subjected to trafficking, racialized people, and people in the developing countries. There is a discussion about this in the contribution to the volume by the archivists, in relation to which keywords and MeSH terms to use when indexing the archive, but pertaining to this volume as a whole, the discursive trajectory that HIV and AIDS have described since the early 1980s provides an interesting problem in nuance: terms that are considered correct today might be anachronistic when applied to a historical material. For instance, the concept of "men who have sex with men," although well established by now, was not an academic term in the 1980s. The choice of words implies an interesting, paradigmatic shift, from a person's identity (as homosexual or gay) to a person's acts, and although some acts (for instance, unprotected anal sex) may transmit the virus, rather than any particular identity, the gay community, founded on such an identity, was, in general, severely hit by the epidemic in its early stages. Accordingly, sometimes it may be more historically correct to use the term gay men, although the material in the archive is indexed with the preferred term men who have sex with men.

Another example is the phrase "people living with HIV." This is the commonly accepted and used term today. However, in the material in the Face of AIDS film archive, people talk about HIV infection, being infected with HIV, being HIV-positive, and having the virus. Actually, in Sweden, there is an HIV support group called "PositHIVa gruppen," placing emphasis on the optimistic and constructive meanings of positive (cf. Ljungcrantz's contribution to this volume). In addition, since the archive covers a span of over thirty years, some footage actually portrays people who are dying of AIDS.

We have tried to be very careful in our use of terminology that might have been perfectly legitimate in the late 1980s and early 1990s but that is considered offensive, condescending, or discriminatory today, balancing the need to be true to the material with the imperative of respectful discourse.

Although the long perspective of the Face of AIDS film archive generates some problems in how to approach the material, this is also a significant strength of the archive. The documentation in the archive captures contemporary moments, like the "AIDS scare" of the mid- to late 1980s, but when we use the material we are looking back in time, with the knowledge and perspectives gained since then. This means that the early material in the archive, in which fear, sadness, anger, frustration, and a sense of injustice and of impending doom for humankind is present, can be watched with the knowledge that at least some of these issues have been resolved. In addition, the development and growth of Hildebrand's own insights into the pandemic during the thirty years he traveled the globe and encountered people to interview and portray is clearly present within the material. For example, in the early footage, Hildebrand does not define himself as an AIDS activist, which he does in the later material. Lately, Hildebrand has also begun returning to interviewees from the early years, showing them clips of themselves and asking them to look back. This retrospective approach shows how Hildebrand himself is using the material in the archive to reflect on the past and his own contribution to the representations of the epidemic and its history, thus reconstructing its meanings. In his own contribution to this volume, Hildebrand also offers a narrative of how and why he began documenting the HIV/AIDS epidemic. This demonstrates in interesting ways how the filmmaker has reinterpreted his own story when, for example compared to statements he made in the 1980s (see Thorsén's contribution to this volume).

A visual history of HIV/AIDS

The historical distance means that new readings and analyses are now possible, which can also be seen in other ways in this anthology. For example, in David Thorsén's chapter, the reception of the film *Crossover: The Global Impact of AIDS* (1988) is closely studied, showing among other things how the film's representation of homosexuality was severely criticized in its contemporaneous context. However, in Tommy Gustafsson's chapter, the film is analyzed in relation to other contexts and in a longer historical perspective, demonstrating how the depiction of homosexual men in the film related to other representations during the era. A strength of the anthology is thus also that different scholars shed light on the material from different perspectives – many of the texts deal with the same material, but offers complementing points of view. Another example of this is how the interview with Australian activist Lyle Taylor is discussed in Anna Sofia Rossholm and Beate Schirrmacher's chapter, and in the chapter by Adam Brenthel and Kristofer Hansson, although using quite different approaches.

We have organized this volume into sections, focusing on different thematic aspects or methodological choices. The first section, Archives, Memories, Histories, contains chapters that deal with the processes of making archives, of creating memories, of testimony and the witnessing of history, and of constructing history from the archival material. It begins with a chapter that explains the legal and ethical challenges involved in making approximately 700 hours of film available online, and how the archive is organized and indexed. In "Face of AIDS: The Making of an Online Archive," Fredrik B. Persson and Martin Kristenson, who work at the library of Karolinska Institutet, discuss the problems they have encountered and how they have solved them.

In "Witnessing AIDS in the Archive," Anna Sofia Rossholm and Beate Schirrmacher examine the Face of AIDS film archive as a net of testimonies of different perspectives and narratives that can convey new insights about HIV and AIDS beyond established facts and mainstream narratives. Drawing upon theories about testimonies and witnessing, Rossholm and Schirrmacher trace how one original interview with Lyle Taylor in Sydney, Australia, in 1988, the early beginnings of Hildebrand's project, has been used in different documentaries later on. The testimonial acts in the archive films and footage are in the analysis framed in a theoretical and historical context of mediated testimonies by comparison with the testimonies of survivor witnesses of other traumas of history (such as the Shoah).

How social memory takes shape is the central question in Cecilia Trenter's contribution, where she reflects on the memory of AIDS in relation to Jan Assman's theory of the transition from a communicative memory to an objectivized culture. "Voices of AIDS: The HIV Virus and the Shaping of a Cultural Memory" addresses the consequences of the remembrance of HIV/AIDS due to the redefinition of AIDS into a treatable condition. The fact that there exists a "before" and an "after" the introduction of antiretroviral therapy is crucial for understanding the representation and memory of HIV/AIDS. By comparing some of Hildebrand's later documentaries with Randy Shilt's famous *And the Band Played On* (1987) and Swedish author and comedian Jonas Gardell's *Don't Ever Wipe Tears without Gloves* (2012–2013), Trenter discusses memory processes and the shaping of a cultural memory.

The section concludes with Daniel Normark's chapter "A Disease on Top of a Disease: People with Hemophilia through the Face of AIDS Film Archive," that revisits the early stage of the tragic U.S. AIDS history. Normark has studied the footage in the archive pertaining to people with hemophilia and constructs a history from the interviews in the material, comparing it with existing historical studies of hemophilia and AIDS. Politically, societally, and medically, people with hemophilia who also suffered from AIDS became instrumental in the development during these early years. Media attention and governmental funding increased. The dual influence of the gay and hemophilia communities helped shape AIDS activism. Furthermore, the search for the cause of the disease and the routes of transmission was narrowed down by the occurrence of AIDS among people with hemophilia.

The second section, Aesthetics, Representations, Narratives, is devoted to analyses of particular films. Hildebrand has used his own footage, at several points through the time period, to make documentary films for various occasions and information purposes. These films are instrumental in understanding Hildebrand's own vision of his project but they are also a part of the archive that has been relatively widely distributed and shown. Tommy Gustafsson looks at "Performativity and Documentary Aesthetics in Staffan Hildebrand's Earliest Conference Films on AIDS in the 1980s," analyzing *AIDS – föreställningar om en verklighet* (1986), and *Crossover: The Global Impact of AIDS* (1988). The main research question of the chapter is how Hildebrand chose to portray an epidemic that had relatively few previous points of cinematic references, especially concerning such things as narrative approach, the use and selection of images and archival footage, the portrayal of people living with HIV, and finally the use of voice-over as a performative element to implement the global impact of the epidemic. The chapter contextualizes Hildebrand's films, partly by a comparison with contemporary films and television series such as *An Early Frost* (1985) and *Dynasty* (1981–1989), but above all by an auteur analysis of Hildebrand's earlier work, both as a documentary filmmaker and as a director of fictional youth films, with the specific aim to develop the theoretical concept of the performative documentary.

In "Disease, Representation, and Activism: *Crossover: The Global Impact of AIDS* (1988) and Its Reverberations," David Thorsén also examines the film *Crossover: The Global Impact of AIDS*, which was presented in 1988 as an international exposé of the ongoing epidemic. Targeting the young, the film toured local schools and was broadcast on television networks all over the world. Praised by many, *Crossover* was also criticized for being tendentious and ignorant, even dangerous to a young audience. In Thorsén's chapter, *Crossover* and its reception are examined as an example of how language, metaphors, and visual and audial imaginary create a particular knowledge of a disease, stressing the importance of the multiple meanings, agents, and strategies in late twentieth-century public health communication.

In "A Positive Positive? Intersectional Analysis of Identification and Counter-identification in three Contemporary HIV Narratives," Desireé Ljungcrantz focuses on the documentary *The Longest Journey Is the Journey Within* (2015), about Steve Sjöquist, an HIV-positive activist, and the autobiographies *Ophelias resa* ("Ophelia's Journey," Larsson and Haanyama Ørum, 2007) and *Mitt positiva liv* ("My Positive Life," Lundstedt and Blankens, 2012). Using the analytical concepts of identifications and counter-identifications, the chapter explores how normativities and deviations are negotiated through portraits of distance and closeness, identificatory narratives, and counter-identifications – relating to a wellness discourse of happiness and positivity normalizing HIV. The analysis of the representations of HIV and people with HIV in three contemporary HIV narratives shows how normative lines are being drawn with the potential to both widen the cultural imaginaries of HIV and reproduce and draw more narrow ideas of who are living with HIV.

Still today, there is a stigma attached to HIV infection. In the third section, Stigma and Trauma, contributors take on a discussion of how stigma and trauma are negotiated in the material in the Face of AIDS film archive. In "Waiting for a Cure: Cultural Perspectives on AIDS in the 1980s," Adam Brenthel and Kristofer Hansson study waiting as a cultural practice in the medical context at the end of the 1980s, with the help of a number of unedited documentary sequences that Hildebrand shot in 1988 together with cameraman Christer Strandell. How is waiting framed in Hildebrand's filming? How is it visually expressed and how does Hildebrand and the people he talks to incarnate it in speech and bodily expressions? Brenthel and Hansson argue that waiting becomes central in the documentary sequences and something that the doctors reflect upon in relation to the questions asked by Hildebrand. In 1988, people were waiting for any new drug that would give life back to young people that had AIDS. People also feared that this emerging infectious disease could spread and escalate. But, above all, people were waiting for death and that burden is reflected by the doctors in the sequences.

Much of Staffan Hildebrand's archive relates to the gay male population, specifically in developing countries, and highlights the vulnerability of gay people living with HIV/AIDS or who are exposed to a high risk of virus transmission because of the structural, interpersonal, and symbolic violence they face. In "Social Suffering as Structural and Symbolic Violence: LGBT Experiences in the Face of AIDS Film Archive," Marco Bacio and Cirus Rinaldi interpret LGBT experiences as evidence of structural, interpersonal, and symbolic violence. Structural violence, especially, is exerted indirectly and systematically by everyone who belongs to a specific social order. Bacio and Rinaldi argue that when we deal with structural violence we must take into account all the dimensions in which oppression can occur. In particular, non-white LGBT groups in developed countries or LGBT minorities in developing countries are at high risk of exposure to violence within their own ethnic group and to vulnerability compared to the wider society.

Mariah Larsson focuses on "Constructions of Safe Sex: Between Desire and Governmentality." Since HIV/AIDS was first identified and conceptualized as an infection without cure and transmitting through various sexual acts, different ways of protection and prevention were prescribed. Perhaps the most significant of these was the idea of "safe sex." With the sexual revolution in the 1960s, and gay liberation following shortly, sexuality had seemed, for a brief time, as freed from the shackles of fear. Now, however, a new threat crept into sexual encounters – most notably within the gay community – and the only way to protect oneself was to adhere to the practices of safe (or safer) sex: abstinence, monogamy, and/or condom use (to be used throughout any sexual act that could lead to the exchange of bodily fluids). Comparing conceptualizations and constructions of safe, safer, and unsafe sex (using these as search terms) in interviews and outtakes made in various countries across the globe from 1988, 1998, and 2008, the chapter asks: How is safe sex defined? Who or what is identified as a threat or the enemy? Where is responsibility placed?

In earlier decades in the twentieth century, educational films about so-called venereal diseases used images of newborn babies covered with sores caused by syphilis as a recurring spectacle. Often, these images were connected to a moral message about how men's sexual relations before or outside marriage could have negative consequences, not only for their own health but for the health of their wives and future children as well. In "Sins of the Fathers? Syphilis, HIV/AIDS, and Innocent Women and Children," Elisabet Björklund uses Hildebrand's films *Women and AIDS* (1990) and *Women at the Frontline* (2008) to examine if similar discourses and representational strategies were used in the case of the HIV epidemic. As many have noted, the discourse around HIV and AIDS early on revolved around ideas of "innocence" and "guilt," and the chapter argues that Hildebrand's films are examples of a feminist discourse in which women and children are to a great extent constructed as innocent victims of the epidemic. As such, there are both similarities and differences between the meanings produced in Hildebrand's films and earlier discourses about syphilis.

The collection concludes with two chapters with a slightly different approach under the heading Activism and Auteurism. In the first one, "Archiving AIDS Activist Video: A Conversation with Jim Hubbard," another HIV/AIDS film archive is portrayed through an interview with its creator. Jim Hubbard, experimental filmmaker and co-founder of the MIX – the New York Queer Experimental Film Festival – has been involved in AIDS activist video since 1987. Together with James Wentzy he helped to build the AIDS Activist Videotape Collection, housed at the New York Public Library. The archival footage from the collection has had an afterlife in various documentaries, after being remediated, among others, in Jim Hubbard's own *United in Anger. A History of ACT UP* (U.S.A., 2012). Therefore, activist video can be said to have a wide impact on the cultural memory of the AIDS epidemic. Together with Sarah Schulman, Hubbard is the founder of the ACT UP Oral History Project, now housed at the

Harvard University Library, which includes interviews with surviving members of the AIDS Coalition to Unleash Power, New York. In the conversation with Dagmar Brunow, he talks about archiving AIDS activist video, about its historical context, its intentions, circulations, and legacies.

In the final chapter of the volume, "Documenting the Journey from AIDS to HIV on Film," Hildebrand himself tells the story of his life and how he came to begin his documentation of the HIV/AIDS epidemic in the late 1980s, highlighting some significant encounters and experiences during his work. Hildebrand reflects on these thirty years and on how he will continue to document the development. As an appendix, Hildebrand has compiled a list of all film projects that have resulted in the Face of AIDS film archive.

Note

1 The history of HIV and AIDS has been chronicled at different points in time during the pandemic, both by scholars and by writers and journalists. A few examples include *And the Band Played On* (Shilts 1987), *AIDS: The Burdens of History* (Fee and Fox 1988), *History of AIDS: Emergence and Origin of a Modern Pandemic* (Grmek 1990), *AIDS at 30: A History* (Harden 2012) and *How to Survive a Plague: The Inside Story of How Citizens and Science Tamed AIDS* (France 2016).

References

Björklund, Elisabet (2012). *The Most Delicate Subject: A History of Sex Education Films in Sweden.* Dissertation. Lund: Lund University.

Bredström, Anna (2008). *Safe Sex, Unsafe Identities: Intersections of "Race," Gender, and Sexuality in Swedish HIV/AIDS Policy*, Dissertation. Linköping University.

Brunow, Dagmar (2017). "Curating Access to Audiovisual Heritage: Cultural Memory and Diversity in European Film Archives," *Image [&] Narrative*, 18(1): 97–110.

Cartwright, Lisa (1995). *Screening the Body: Tracing Medicine's Visual Culture.* Minneapolis, MN: University of Minnesota Press.

Eberwein, Robert (1999). *Sex Ed: Film, Video, and the Framework of Desire*, New Brunswick, NJ, and London: Rutgers University Press.

Engh, Sunniva (2009). "The Conscience of the World?: Swedish and Norwegian Provision of Development Aid," *Itinerario*, 33(2) (Scandinavian Colonialism): 65–82.

Fee, Elizabeth and Daniel M. Fox, eds. (1988). *AIDS: The Burdens of History.* Berkeley, CA: University of California Press.

France, David (2016). *How to Survive a Plague: The Inside Story of How Citizens and Science Tamed AIDS.* London: Picador.

Friedman, Lester D., ed. (2004). *Cultural Sutures: Medicine and Media.* Durham, NC, and London: Duke University Press.

Gardell, Jonas (2012). *Torka aldrig tårar utan handskar. 1, Kärleken.* Stockholm: Norstedt.

Gardell, Jonas (2013). *Torka aldrig tårar utan handskar. 2, Sjukdomen.* Stockholm: Norstedt.

Gardell, Jonas (2013). *Torka aldrig tårar utan handskar. 3, Döden.* Stockholm: Norstedt.

Griffin, Gabriele (2000). *Representations of HIV/AIDS – Visibility Blue/s.* Manchester and New York: Manchester University Press.

Grmek, Mirko (1990). *History of AIDS: Emergence and Origin of a Modern Pandemic*, translated from French by Russell C. Maulitz and Jacalyn Duffin. Princeton, NJ: Princeton University Press (originally published as *Historire du sida: Début et origine d'un pandemic actuelle*, 1989).

Hallas, Roger (2009). *Reframing Bodies: AIDS, Bearing Witness, and the Queer Moving Image*. Durham, NC: Duke University Press.

Harden, Victoria Angela (2012). *AIDS at 30: A History*. 1st ed. Washington, DC: Potomac.

Hart, Kylo-Patrick R. (2000). *The AIDS Movie – Representing a Pandemic in Film and Television*. New York, London, and Oxford: Haworth.

Henriksson, Benny (1988). *Social Democracy or Societal Control: A Critical Analysis of Swedish AIDS Policy*. Stockholm: Institute for Social Policy [Institutet för sociala studier].

Henriksson, Benny (1995). *Risk Factor Love: Homosexuality, Sexual Interaction and HIV Prevention*. Dissertation. Gothenburg University.

Henriksson, Benny and Hasse Ytterberg (1992). "Sweden: The Power of the Moral(istic) Left," in David L. Kirp and Ronald Bayer (eds.), *AIDS in the Industrialized Democracies: Passions, Politics, and Policies*, 317–338. New Brunswick, NJ: Rutgers University Press.

Juhasz, Alexandra (1995). *AIDS TV: Identity, Community, and Alternative Video*. Durham, NC, and London: Duke University Press.

Lennerhed, Lena (1994). *Frihet att njuta: sexualdebatten i Sverige på 1960-talet*. Dissertation. Stockholm: Norstedts.

Ljung, Anna (2001). *Bortom oskuldens tid – en etnologisk studie av moral, trygghet och otrygghet i skuggan av hiv*. Dissertation. Uppsala: Uppsala University.

McKinnon, Kenneth (1992). *The Politics of Popular Representation – Reagan, Thatcher, AIDS, and the Movies*. Rutherford, Madison, and Teaneck, NJ: Fairleigh Dickinson University Press.

Milliken, Christie (2003). *Generation Sex: Reconfiguring Sexual Citizenship in Educational Film and Video*. Dissertation. University of Southern California.

Noaks Ark (2017). *HIV-rapporten*, http://noaksark.org/wp-content/uploads/2017/09/Hivrapporten_sept-2017-.pdf, last accessed October 30, 2017.

Ostherr, Kirsten (2013). *Medical Visions: Producing the Patient through Film, Television, and Imaging Technologies*. Oxford: Oxford University Press.

Patton, Cindy (1990). *Inventing AIDS*. New York and London: Routledge.

Reagan, Leslie J., Nancy Tomes, and Paula A.Treichler, eds. (2008 [2007]). *Medicine's Moving Pictures: Medicine, Health, and Bodies in American Film and Television*. Rochester, NY: University of Rochester Press.

Shilts, Randy (1987). *And the Band Played On: Politics, People, and the AIDS Epidemic*. New York: St. Martin's Press.

Snickars, Pelle and Patrick Vonderau, eds. (2009). *The YouTube Reader*. Stockholm: KB.

Sontag, Susan (1990 [1977, 1988]). *Illness as Metaphor and AIDS and Its Metaphors*. New York: Picador.

Thorsén, David (2013). *Den svenska aidsepidemin – ankomst, bemötande, innebörd*. Dissertation. Uppsala: Acta Universitatis Upsaliensis, Uppsala Studies in History of Ideas 44.

Treichler, Paula A. (1999). *How to Have Theory in an Epidemic – Cultural Chronicles of AIDS*. Durham, NC, and London: Duke University Press.

UNAIDS (2017). *UNAIDS Data 2017*, www.unaids.org/en/resources/documents/2017/2017_data_book, last accessed November 24, 2017.

Watney, Simon (1997 [1987]). *Policing Desire: Pornography, AIDS, and the Media*. 3rd ed. London: Cassell.

Films and TV productions

Armfield, Neil, *Holding the Man* (2015).
Campillo, Robin, *120 BPM* (2017).
Cardone, Daniel F., *Desert Migration* (2015).
Dynasty (1981–1989).
Erman, John, *An Early Frost* (1985).
France, David, *How to Survive a Plague* (2012).
Hildebrand, Staffan, *AIDS – föreställningar om en verklighet* (1986).
Hildebrand, Staffan, *Crossover: The Global Impact of AIDS* (1988).
Hildebrand, Staffan, *Women and AIDS* (1990).
Hildebrand, Staffan, *Women at the Frontline* (2008).
Hildebrand, Staffan, *The Longest Journey Is the Journey Within* (2015).
Hubbard, Jim, *United in Anger. A History of ACT UP* (2012).
Kaijser, Simon, *Don't Ever Wipe Tears without Gloves/Torka aldrig tårar utan handskar* (2012).
Nichols, Mike, *Angels in America* (2003).
Vallée, Jean-Marc, *Dallas Buyers Club* (2013).
Weissman, David and Bill Weber, *We Were Here* (2011).

Part I

Archives, memories, histories

1 Face of AIDS

The making of an online archive

Martin Kristenson and Fredrik B. Persson

Introduction[1]

For more than thirty years, starting in 1986, film director and journalist Staffan Hildebrand has documented the global AIDS epidemic (Wolfson 2004). He has made films for fifty AIDS conferences and produced about 700 hours of footage from more than forty countries. The archive includes complete documentaries as well as unedited raw material. Hildebrand has interviewed scientists, AIDS activists, people living with HIV, people who inject drugs, sex workers and many others with experience of HIV and AIDS. He has filmed in laboratories and at conferences, in hospitals and on the street. The Face of AIDS (FoA) project covers three decades of HIV and AIDS history from many different perspectives, and is invaluable not only for medical historians but also for film scholars, political scientists, sociologists and others interested in issues related to HIV and AIDS.

In the spring of 2013, all the films were digitized, and on 18 September the same year the entire archive was handed over to Karolinska Institutet (KI). The archive also contained metadata about time, location, details of the persons involved and in many cases a short description of the content and context of the film.

Shortly after the handover to KI, a project group was formed at Karolinska Institutet University Library (KIB) with the objective of securing the material for the future and making it accessible, mainly for research and teaching but to a limited extent also to the general public.

The first thing we did in the project group was to study other online film archives. We also talked to representatives from a couple of Swedish film archives, especially Filmarkivet.se, a joint project for Swedish shorts, non-fiction films, newsreels and commercials initiated by the Swedish Film Institute and the National Library of Sweden. They gave us advice, mostly on technical details and editorial issues but also on metadata and indexing. We also found that we had a lot to learn from studying Shoah Foundation Visual History Archive, both in the way they describe and categorize their films and in the way they handle integrity questions and sensitive content.

In addition to the technical challenge of building a searchable online archive of such a comprehensive material, the project faced difficult questions: On what legal and ethical conditions is it possible for a medical university to publish and make this type of film archive available online? And how should journalistic films be described in a medical academic context?

Legal and ethical issues

When we first started working with the archive, we were not aware of the sensitive nature of some of the films. After all, Hildebrand's documentaries had been shown without problems at AIDS conferences, seminars and film festivals and on television channels all over the world. However, we soon realized that the issue was more complicated than we thought. First, since a large number of the documentaries were filmed long before the Internet was widely accessible, the participants could not have foreseen how the Web would dramatically change film distribution. They may have agreed for a film to be screened once but not to be available globally at any time. An interviewee may also have a new life situation and not want to be reminded of the past.

Pictures of dying AIDS patients and children, who often have not had a chance to agree to being filmed, presented another complication for the archive. Many AIDS patients freely give interviews in their hospital beds, but in several other cases the camera sweeps across the ward, recording people too sick to pay any attention.

Furthermore, some of the unedited footage contains material that was not supposed to be made public. Examples of this are comments made by participants unaware of the camera being on or an extreme close-up of an interviewee's face. In a few cases, people wanting to be anonymous for a documentary are nevertheless

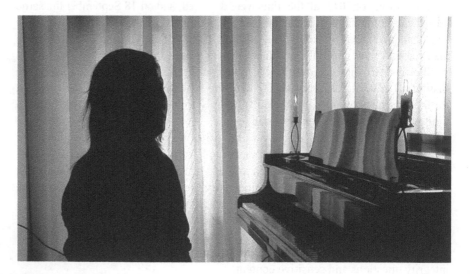

Figure 1.1 Anonymous woman. *Vi och dom.*
Source: Hildebrand, 2005.

shown and named in the unedited footage. When we looked through the archive in more detail, we encountered more films that needed to be discussed thoroughly, for example:

- In one film from 2006, a young woman is interviewed about her HIV status and her activist work with young people. At first, we found nothing problematic with this film – it had been shown at a big AIDS conference – but then we read a comment in the metadata saying that the woman had agreed to participate in the film on the condition that it would only be shown at the AIDS conference. We later discovered that she openly discusses her HIV status when lecturing in front of a smaller audience but not when she is interviewed for television or for a documentary film. Consequently, she also appeared anonymously in an earlier documentary from 2005.
- In an interview made in 1989, a young woman from a Western country talks openly about living with HIV. While doing research on the archive's history, we found an interview which she gave for a Swedish newspaper. She had come to Sweden to promote the film and appeared with her photo and real name, but told the reporter that she would never agree to do that in her homeland. Indeed, her family did not know of her HIV status. In those days, you could still choose to be open in one country and anonymous in another. However, with the development of the Internet, this is now impossible.
- There is also some footage of people who are not fully conscious. In 1998, the FoA team joined two social workers on their nightly walk around a large Eastern European city, where they met and spoke to a 16-year-old girl who injected drugs. She answered their questions but did not seem to be aware of the camera being on.
- For the most part, interviews conducted with randomly selected people on the street, "vox populi", did not present any problem, but some of them did. For example, the FoA archive contains an interview from 1988 with two Western tourists in the Philippines. They are having a night out at nightclubs, bars and massage parlours, and do not appear to reflect on their words being recorded. In another film, a 14-year-old orphan girl in an African country was interviewed in 1998. Her parents died of AIDS and she took care of her five siblings. In the film, we see her preparing food for her family. Since she was a child at the time, we first thought the film could not be made public, but we had second thoughts when we found out that the girl at the same time had spoken at an AIDS conference and that her speech was reported in articles afterwards. She is also featured in one of Hildebrand's earlier documentaries.
- Since fighting stigma is an important part of the HIV response, many activists chose to be open about their HIV status. Would it be disrespectful to anonymize them or are there instances when that would be more appropriate? Considering an activist giving television interviews or lectures at International AIDS Conferences may seem unproblematic, but what about

an openly gay activist living in a country with strict anti-gay laws? Or, for that matter, an activist working in a small community, open with his or her HIV status but not a public figure? What is our responsibility here?

• In a film from 1988, an AIDS activist from the organization ACT UP and her husband are interviewed about their HIV diagnoses and their relationship as a married couple. Their small HIV-negative daughter is seen throughout the film. As an activist, the woman wanted to share her story, but the film also contains privacy-sensitive information. Which one of these considerations should be given the greatest importance?

Relevant legislation

Since Hildebrand worked as a news reporter and documentary filmmaker, one can argue that his work for the FoA archive should be made publicly available. However, what would be appropriate to publish for the general public in one context, for example a newspaper, is not necessarily appropriate in the domain of a medical university.

Owing to the fact that Hildebrand's films represent both journalistic work and documentation intended for scientific use, different laws apply depending on how the archive is used – as a resource for public information or as a database for scholarly research. When the film material is made available on the Internet for the benefit of the general public, one has to consider the Swedish Personal Data Act (SFS 1998:204), whereas when the film archive is made available to researchers one has to consider the Swedish Act Concerning the Ethical Review of Research Involving Humans (SFS 2003:460). The Swedish Personal Data Act is aimed at preventing the violation of personal integrity by the processing of personal data. There are no specific rules regarding publication on the Internet in the Act. Publishing personal information on websites is allowed as long as it is not in an offensive context. What should be considered a violation is difficult to define in a simple principle as it depends on the context (The Ministry of Justice 2006). Since the context is not offensive in this case, it would seem that the Swedish Personal Data Act does not limit public access to the archive. Furthermore, works of journalistic and artistic nature are protected by the laws regulating freedom of speech and freedom of the press.

It can be argued that when the participants agreed to be interviewed they also publicly announced their statements in a journalistic context, unless otherwise agreed. This is particularly true regarding interviews conducted with people who represent an organization or act in their professional roles. Making journalistic film clips like these available for the purpose of a public archive should fall outside the limitation of the Swedish Personal Data Act.

However, a special part of the Act prohibits the processing of personal data if it contains any of the following, so-called privacy-sensitive data concerning:

• Race or ethnicity
• Political opinions

- Religious or philosophical beliefs
- Membership of trade unions
- Information about health and sexual life.

Exceptions from this rule apply if the person in question clearly publicized the information. There are several examples of activists in the archive that openly disclose their HIV status during the interviews. Should this information be considered privacy-sensitive? Probably not, but it may be so when the film clips are viewed as research data.

Legislation and ethical recommendations relevant to the scientific application of the FoA archive usually refer to the idea of good research practice. As the Swedish Research Council outlines in one of its publications (Swedish Research Council 1:2005), research ethics are not static – as new material and methods evolve the research community faces new questions and has to find a reasonable balance between various interests.

In 2004, a law dealing with ethical vetting of research that involves humans was passed in Sweden. The purpose of the law is to protect the individual and the respect for human dignity in research. It encompasses research involving living persons but it also covers such areas as research on the deceased, biological material from people and research that involves privacy-sensitive personal data. In the law there are special rules which apply to research methods that have an obvious risk to harm the individual either physically or mentally. The vetting is conducted by the Central Ethical Review Board in Sweden, which approves applications from researchers.

Making the archive available to users

Our ambition has always been to keep the archive as open as possible. However, after considering the legal and ethical issues outlined above, we realized that a completely open archive would not be possible. Following the example of other online film archives (Shoah Foundation Visual History Archive and the Red Cross Audiovisual Archive), we decided to make the FoA archive available on three levels. In assigning films to the different levels, our goal was to restrict availability only when absolutely necessary:

> **Level 1 (public access)**: Films of a public nature (lectures, demonstrations, interviews etc.), accessible on the FoA website. This includes a searchable selection of documentaries and edited footage from the archive. At the time of writing, there are about 300 publicly available films, but we are adding more on a regular basis. The public website is also provided with a disclaimer, giving people appearing in the films an opportunity to request the removal of the content and personal information. For publicly available documentaries, we have decided to pixelate the faces of people in vulnerable situations (people who inject drugs, sex workers, children, gay activists from countries with strict anti-gay laws etc.).

Level 2 (partial access): In a password-protected part of the website, trusted users – researchers, teachers and students working on an essay or project linked to a higher education institution – can search the full archive index with the exception of privacy-sensitive personal data. In addition, films of a public nature not yet adapted for Level 1 can be viewed at this level. Researchers can make request for films not yet manually checked to be made available at Level 2. The FoA staff will then review the film and, if possible, make it available. To gain access to Level 2, all users need to sign an agreement regarding professional secrecy of the archives content. We are regularly adding more (not privacy-sensitive) films to this level.

Level 3 (full access): Trusted users can gain access to the full FoA archive, all of the footage and the full index, in the special viewing room that has been prepared at KIB. This means that users must come to the library to access the film archive. Access to Level 3 can be given to researchers/ research groups with approval from the Swedish Ethical Review Board, a project description and an approval from KIB. In addition, teachers and students working on an essay or project affiliated with higher education at KI can be given access to Level 3 after an approval from KIB. Their institution has to demonstrate that there are ethical routines in place for handling privacy-sensitive material. In cases where researchers need access to Level 3 in order to get a better understanding of the content of the archive in preparation for their research project, the library can grant temporary access. All users of Level 3 have to sign an agreement regarding professional secrecy of the archive's content.

With the decision to divide the archive into three levels, we could go ahead and sort the individual films. To return to the examples under the legal and ethical issues section above, we found that only a few films could be made public:

- Regarding the activist who had agreed to only one screening of the film, we decided that it would be a violation of the agreement with the woman if we did not conceal her face. Therefore, she is anonymized in all versions of the film, even at Level 3.
- The footage of the woman interviewed in a Swedish newspaper and the girl who injected drugs were both categorized as Level 3.
- The documentary in which the two tourists appear is made available at Level 1, but with pixilated faces. The unedited film clip with them is only available on Level 3.
- In view of the fact that the story of the orphan girl is already public, and told by herself at an International AIDS Conference, we decided not to anonymize her.
- After some discussion, we came to the conclusion that it would be absurd to anonymize well-known activists interviewed in the archive. It would probably injure their dignity and counter their objective by making their

stories anonymous. An exception from this rule is footage with openly gay activists in countries with anti-gay laws, or others who risk persecution in their home countries. These films are categorized as Level 3. Films with lesser-known activists will be decided from case to case. If possible, we try to contact them before we make a decision. As for the ACT UP activist, we decided to make the interview available on Level 1. Although she discloses privacy-sensitive information in the film, her decision as an AIDS activist to share her story was crucial in this case.

Indexing the archive

Indexing film – as opposed to scientific articles – has its own special conditions. Since the FoA archive largely consists of unedited film footage (location shots, spontaneous conversations and improvisations), it was a great challenge to organize the material and make it searchable. The films' breadth of content – from scientific lectures to everyday reflections – made the choice of indexing terms particularly difficult. The goal was also to make the archive useful for scientists as well as laymen, and indexing had therefore to be made at a level that worked for both groups.

Our starting point was the metadata handed over along with the film material. The basic facts of the films in the archive – dates, locations, names, summaries etc. – were listed in an Excel file, without which we could not have done any indexing at all. We also realized the value of Hildebrand's unique knowledge and asked him to put as much as possible about the films in writing – memories, anecdotes, biographies. In addition to this, we filmed forty short interviews with Hildebrand in which he tells background stories about specific films. In the future, it is also our intention to interview some of his collaborators.

The indexing of the archive's 700 hours of film was done in two steps. First, we divided the material into twelve broad categories, indicating the main themes of the film: "Treatment and care", "Personal Stories", "Science/Research", "Activism & NGOs", "Stigma" etc. Each category was provided with a brief description to clarify what type of films were included. In view of the fact that many films had more than one theme, especially the unedited footage, it was decided that a film could be included in a maximum of three categories.

For a more detailed description of specific content in each film, we decided to use Medical Subject Headings (MeSH), the controlled vocabulary thesaurus produced by the National Library of Medicine. This was an obvious choice, since there are more than 27,000 descriptors in MeSH and the thesaurus is used by the world's largest medical database MEDLINE/PubMed and many other medical databases.

However, we discovered that MeSH was not sufficient to describe the documentaries and unedited footage included in the archive. We needed to create our own thesaurus as a complement to MeSH. At the moment, we have about ninety keywords, ranging from the artwork "AIDS Memorial Quilt" and the district "Zona Rosa" in Mexico City to "Hip Hop", "Patient Zero" and "Pride festivals". The keywords also provide an easier way to search the archive for laymen and other users not used to MeSH. For the sake of clarity, we have sometimes combined MeSH terms with keywords. For instance, the term "AIDS Serodiagnosis" may not be understood by everyone, and is therefore complemented with the keyword "HIV Tests". In the same way, the MeSH term "Infectious Disease Transmission, Vertical" is always combined with the keyword "Mother-To-Child Transmission (MTCT)".

Hildebrand's films have often been shot for specific purposes, such as conferences, scientific meetings and information campaigns. Since they do not have the strict structure of a scientific article, there were difficulties in applying MeSH terms to them. An interview may cover several topics, although many of them are discussed only for a few minutes or less. Therefore, we had to decide for how long an interviewee must speak on a topic – and how detailed the discussion should be – for it to be indexed. There was no given answer, but our main focus was to provide relevant search results for our users.

One question asked by researchers was if Hildebrand followed a scientific method in conducting his interviews. The answer is no – as mentioned earlier, Hildebrand is a documentary filmmaker, and all the films in the archive are journalistic works. However, going through the films, we found that Hildebrand and his team often have returned to certain questions and discussions in their interviews. We thought that researchers might be interested in identifying these questions in order to compare how they have been answered in different places and/ or periods of time. We compiled a list of the most common questions, and the MeSH terms/keywords they had been indexed with. For instance:

- "How can you change the power structure between men and women?" (MeSH: Sexism).
- "Are you an optimist?"/"What do you think about the future?" (Keyword: Future Perspectives).
- "There is a lot of discussion about ending AIDS. As a scientist, how do you see it?" (Keyword: Ending AIDS, MeSH: Disease Eradication).

Using this list, it is also possible to see if some questions have been more frequently asked at certain times. For example, the question whether "AIDS is an answer from Nature" (MeSH: Nature) was almost exclusively asked in 1988, while the question of "ending AIDS" becomes more common in the 2000s.

From 2011 and onwards, Hildebrand made a series of follow-up interviews with people he met and filmed the years before. In these interviews, the interviewees describe their reactions on seeing the old film clips and comment on what has happened since then. These films are indexed as "Follow-Up Interview".

Choosing appropriate terminology

The terms used to describe the HIV epidemic have changed considerably in the thirty-year period that the FoA archive films span. In the early days of AIDS, terms like "gay cancer" or "gay plague" were not uncommon. There was also talk of "high-risk groups", "AIDS victims" etc., concepts which pointed out certain groups in society and implicitly saw the disease as a punishment. Consequently, it was important for us to find correct terms, ones that are not stigmatizing or may be perceived as excluding. From the start, we decided to use the terms included in the terminology guide issued by the Joint United Nations Programme on HIV and AIDS (UNAIDS) along with the MeSH thesaurus. There were two problems with this, as we soon found out.

First, UNAIDS and MeSH do not always agree on what terms to use. For instance, UNAIDS recommends not using the term "prostitution", as it denotes value judgement (UNAIDS 2015), but at the time we started indexing it was still a MeSH term. We decided to go both ways and follow UNAIDS's recommendations in our own texts and background material but use MeSH terms when indexing, even if they collided with UNAIDS's recommendations. In this case, the problem was solved when the MeSH term "prostitution" was changed to "sex work" in 2017.

Second, we found that our choices sometimes would be controversial no matter what terms we settled for. Again, "sex worker" is a case in point. Many people consider this term a euphemism for sexual exploitation and criminal activity. To quote an open letter to the Associated Press, signed by 300 organizations and activists in 2014, the term was "invented by the sex industry and its supporters in order to legitimize prostitution as a legal and acceptable form of work and conceal its harm to those exploited in the commercial sex trade" (Unizon 2017).

On the other hand, advocates of the term argue that "sex worker" is non-judgemental and destigmatizing, and is also a way to recognize the legal rights of persons in the sex industry. In 2016, Amnesty International adopted a policy for the rights of sex workers, declaring that the organization neither supports nor condemns commercial sex: "But we do strongly condemn human rights abuses committed against people who sell sex and the discrimination they face; and we believe decriminalization is one important step towards addressing that" (Amnesty International 2017).

In the end, since the FoA archive takes no position on this issue, we decided to use UNAIDS Terminology Guide and always refer to its recommendations. Finally, we turned to a number of Swedish AIDS organizations and let them comment critically on the FoA website. We only received one objection – the use of a slash in "HIV/AIDS". It was said that the terms should be used separately to avoid confusion between HIV (a virus) and AIDS (a clinical diagnosis).

Ideas for future development of the archive

In many aspects, the archive now meets the vision presented by two researchers at KI in an article in 2011:

> The vision for the archive is the development of a digitally accessible, online film archive of HIV/AIDS. The archive represents a unique visual

26   *Martin Kristenson and Fredrik B. Persson*

education, research and information tool, which documents how the AIDS pandemic and the response to it have evolved over time around the world.

(Albert and Chiodi 2011: 503)

We are currently discussing how we can develop the archive further in this direction and make it more dynamic and relevant for public debate.

At the moment, the only background material we have in the archive is the comments provided by Hildebrand himself. We still have to decide how to make good use of all of his writings on the subject. In the future, we hope to broaden the archive by inviting researchers, journalists and others to contribute essays and analyses.

We also think it is important to use the FoA archive films to give a historical perspective on current HIV issues. For instance, it would have been a good idea if we could have highlighted film clips on the so-called "Patient Zero" when new findings about him were published in 2016 (Worobey *et al.* 2016: 98–101). We could also make selections from the archive and present them in conjunction with World AIDS Day, the International AIDS Conferences and other HIV-related events. For this purpose, we plan to use social media in some way – e.g. Twitter and Facebook.

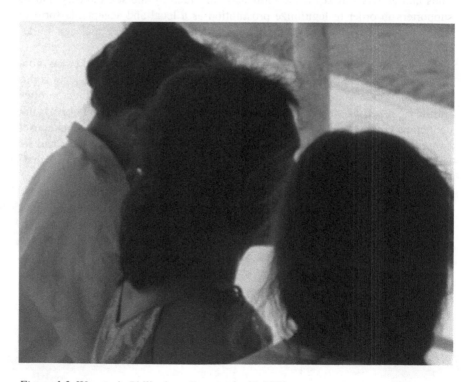

Figure 1.2 Women in Philippines diagnosed with HIV.
Source: Archive ID 1988_76.

Another idea is to have recurrent "virtual exhibitions" on the website, as used by the television history portal EUscreen and Filmarkivet.se, where a few films from the archive are selected to shed light on a particular theme (such as "Cambodia", "Stigma", "Women and AIDS" etc.). By juxtaposing films from various countries and environments, as well as different periods of time, new knowledge and insights can be gained.

We are also interested in a closer collaboration with the scholarly community and with educational institutions. Our work on this anthology with Linnaeus University is a first step in that direction.

In addition, we have also discussed the possibility to include documentary films from other sources than the FoA project and make the archive a virtual museum on HIV and AIDS.

In conclusion, the FoA film archive is a unique visual history of a global epidemic. It chronicles three decades of the virus, from the early years until today, through triumphs and defeats, joy and sorrow, and with new films still being added to the archive. In an interview made for the archive in 2002, the leading biomedical researcher Robert C. Gallo (director and co-founder of the Institute of Human Virology) concluded that it "seems evident, but maybe it needs to be said, that the documentation of the epidemic is extremely important. Otherwise, in the course of time, people will forget and we shall have mythology and not the truth" (Gallo 2002).

Note

1 We would like to thank Glenn Haya and Sofia Samuelsson for their advice and comments on our chapter.

References

Albert, J. and F. Chiodi (2011). "Towards a World Free from HIV and AIDS?" *Journal of Internal Medicine*, 270(6): 502–508. doi:10.1111/j.1365–2796.2011.02453.x.

Amnesty International (2017). *Q&A: Policy to Protect the Human Rights of Sex Workers*, www.amnesty.org/en/qa-policy-to-protect-the-human-rights-of-sex-workers, last accessed 11 April 2017.

Gallo, R. (2002). France 2002, Archive ID: 2002_14. *Face of AIDS Film Archive*. http://faceofaids.ki.se/archive/2002-14, last accessed 11 April 2017.

The Ministry of Justice. *Personal Data Protection – Information on the Personal Data Act* [brochure], www.regeringen.se/contentassets/87382a7887764e9995db186244b557 e4/personal-data-protection (4th revised ed. 2006).

SFS 1998:204. The Swedish Personal Data Act. Stockholm: The Ministry of Justice.

SFS 2003:460. The Ethical Review Act. Stockholm: The Ministry of Education and Research.

Swedish Research Council. (2011). *Good Research Practice* (Report 3:2011). Stockholm, https://publikationer.vr.se/produkt/good-research-practice, last accessed 29 September 2017.

UNAIDS (2011). *Terminology Guide*, www.unaids.org/sites/default/files/media_asset/ JC2118_terminology-guidelines_en_1.pdf, last accessed 29 September 2017.

UNAIDS   (2015).   *Terminology   Guide*,   www.unaids.org/sites/default/files/media_
    asset/2015_terminology_guidelines_en.pdf, last accessed 29 September 2017.
Unizon (2017). *Open Letter to AP from 300 Organizations and Activists*, http://unizon.se/
    sites/default/files/media/_ppet_brev_ap_31_oct_2014_51389.pdf,   last   accessed   11
    April 2017.
Wolfson, W. (2004). "Profile – Staffan Hildebrand: Filmmaker Who Charts the Spread of
    AIDS", *The Lancet*, 364: 1931, www.thelancet.com/pdfs/journals/lancet/PIIS014067
    3604174990.pdf.
Worobey, M., T.D. Watts, R.A. McKay, M.A. Suchard, T. Granade, D.E. Teuwen, B.A.
    Koblin, W. Heneine, P. Lemey and H.W. Jaffe (2016). "1970s and 'Patient 0' HIV-1
    Genomes Illuminate Early HIV/AIDS History in North America", *Nature*, 539(7627):
    98–101. doi:10.1038/nature19827.

2 Witnessing AIDS in the archive

Anna Sofia Rossholm and Beate Schirrmacher

In 1999, Paula A. Treichler stated that the story of HIV and AIDS "remains untold" (Treichler 1999: 204). If this is still an accurate statement, it is not because there are few films, documentaries, and books on the subject of HIV and AIDS but because the experiences of the epidemic generally seem to be either lost in stereotypes and melodramatic narratives about victims and survivors or shared only in small cultural circles and communities.

Can new media forms, such as the digital archive, provide a platform that bridges the gap between existing narratives and enables new perspectives on HIV and AIDS? The Face of AIDS film archive does not offer anything that can be considered to be a coherent story but rather a patchwork of testimonies that is lacking a unifying narrative. In this chapter, we suggest that only such a plurality and heterogeneous mix of different perspectives and narratives has the potential to convey new insights about HIV and AIDS that go beyond established facts and mainstream narratives.

We will thus approach the Face of AIDS film archive from the perspective of testimony and the act of witnessing. In the archive, different narratives both explicitly testify and implicitly bear witness to experiences and changing perspectives throughout the history of HIV and AIDS – from the 1980s until today. Patients, relatives, doctors, scientists, and activists across different periods and cultural and social contexts share subjective, often personal, experiences of HIV and AIDS. Rather than searching for one convincing narrative, we approached the archive by asking what its sprawling and heterogeneous material might bear witness to. Thus, we focused not only on what is said but asked how specific stories relate to the context provided by the archive. What does each add to our understanding of HIV and AIDS? This perspective enables us to relate heterogeneous narratives to one another, allowing seemingly digressive narratives and leftover footage to be studied in the light of the corpus of edited material and clearly verbalised testimonies. Thus, we can highlight how the Face of AIDS film archive increases our understanding of the epidemic as an unfolding process.

Many films in the archive describe traumatic experiences, and as such share similarities with the testimonies of survivor witnesses of other historical traumas (such as the Shoah). Understanding the challenge faced by survivors – putting into words extremely traumatic experiences – was therefore an important starting point in approaching interviews with patients with AIDS. In contrast to most other forms of witnessing, however, the epidemic is ongoing while being documented affecting the ways in which it can be witnessed.

This chapter discusses these complex relations based on the case study of the thirty-minute interview with Lyle Taylor, a dying AIDS patient, conducted in Sydney in 1988 – one of the earliest interviews in the Face of AIDS film archive. It is also the first interview that Staffan Hildebrand conducted with a person dying from AIDS and, notably, recurs in a variety of his documentary films produced between the late 1980s and 2010s. An analysis of the trajectory of the film footage across the archive shows that the reframing and editing of a film excerpt may change what it testifies to. Approaching the raw footage from the perspective of witnessing highlights how expressing subjectivity can be understood in relation to the experience of AIDS. In the following, we begin by delineating some theoretical perspectives on witnessing, testimony, and representation, and continue with analysis of the documentaries in which the interview with Lyle Taylor is featured. We discuss the raw footage of the interview towards the end of the chapter.

Giving testimony and bearing witness

Witnesses verbalise their perceptions and experiences to an audience that does not necessarily share their experience. Listening to witnesses is thus a way of gaining knowledge beyond one's own experience. This transfer of knowledge, however, is "fragile" (Peters 2001: 710), as it builds on certain tensions between body and word, subjectivity and objectivity (Assmann 2007; Krämer 2015: 144–164).

Witnessing relates verbal testimony to bodily presence and depends on trust between witness and audience. The bodily presence of a witness in front of an audience links the present moment to an event in the past. This "bodily basis of witnessing" (Peters 2001: 712) bears witness; it confirms or may undermine a verbal testimony. The witness also has to be a reliable person, as the audience has to trust the witness. To listen to a witness is acknowledging their social status, wherein the witness "vouches for his word with his character" (Krämer 2015: 148).

Witnessing relates subjective experience and memory to the objectivity of facts, evidence, and established knowledge. The legal witness in court is thus asked to focus on perception and refrain from subjective evaluation, as memories or perceptions are used to establish evidence (Krämer 2015: 146; see also Peters 2001: 711–717). A contemporary witness in a documentary, on the other hand, is explicitly asked to contribute with subjective memories of a particular event in the past, which are used to expand our knowledge of how historical events were experienced.

Witnessing provides new knowledge but also relates to what is already known – "the community's shared perception of reality, common sense" (Engdahl 2002: 8).

Testimonies are often used to increase the credibility of a certain narrative, be it that of the prosecution in court or a documentary's overarching story. The verbal testimony of a traumatic experience, however, strives to verbalise an experience that deviates from and perhaps contradicts common sense (Ibid.), and deals with events that may even resist verbalisation.

In witnessing traumatic experiences, the tensions between a verbal testimony and what it might bear witness to are pushed to the limits. Survivors of atrocities such as the Shoah invert and "fracture" basic forms of witnessing (Krämer 2015: 157; see also Baer 2000; Assmann 2007; Elm and Kößler 2007), as they are both victims of atrocities and witnesses of the deaths of others. Thus, survivors will always speak on behalf of those victims who died (Englund 2002: 53; Levi 1988: 64). Their testimony also possesses credibility owing to the closeness to pain and death, and does not depend on but instead restores and acknowledges, social identity, which they have been made bereft of by death and pain (Krämer 2015: 158–159).

The subjective experience of pain and lethal threat is the core of every survivor testimony, and may not be possible to fully express in words. Survivor testimonies may therefore lack coherence and appear to be dysfunctional. As fragmented narratives, they may bear witness rather than verbally testify to the impact of trauma. Such a testimony does not corroborate and cannot be contained within an overarching narrative; rather, a dysfunctional, fragmentary narrative of a survivor bears witness to an experience that is impossible create a logical and structured account of.

If verbal testimony is distorted by the impact of trauma, the audience must provide the coherence that the witness cannot provide by acting as secondary witnesses (Baer 2000: 19–20). In the very act of listening, they acknowledge the fact that the dysfunctional verbal testimony bears witness to the extent of the trauma. This audience does not have to be co-present in order to provide the necessary recognition and coherence, however, and literature, art, and film can act as an "intellectual witness", mediating testimony in a way that acknowledges the difficulties inherent in expressing pain and trauma (Hartman 2000: 35–52). Intellectual witnessing thus mediates the responsibility and moral impetus of a co-present audience to a secondary one (Baer 2000: 24).

Witnessing HIV and AIDS

The AIDS epidemic has been documented and witnessed not as an event of the past but as a still-unfolding phenomenon. In the archive, there are many accounts of contemporary witnesses that look back on past events and are thus able to verbalise and reflect on their experiences. Other interviews in the archive, however, reflect on the present situation and bear witness to the process of struggling with uncertainty and the presence of AIDS as a lethal threat. Here, temporal distance, which characterises many other forms of witnessing, is lacking. This is most acutely felt in the interviews conducted with patients suffering with AIDS in the 1980s. They were not interviewed as survivors of atrocities; rather, they were victims that speak as witnesses while still subject to lethal threat. However, unlike the victims of the Shoah or a sudden catastrophic event, they are victims who are able to speak out, significantly shifting their roles as witnesses.

Patients with AIDS in the 1980s who were interviewed testified at the time in which they were living a traumatic situation – while in pain, while expecting death. They are thus both moribund victims and eyewitnesses. Visually, they are often presented as victimised, othered bodies. When they are interviewed, however, the shapes of their bodies no longer victimise them, as it instead forms the basis of their witnessing. In speaking and sharing their experiences, they are witnesses and thus speak as socially respected individuals. To the survivor, the act of witnessing restores a bereft subjectivity; to the patient with AIDS, the act of witnessing keeps their subjectivity present, which – when speaking – is threatened by death.

When an individual speaks under lethal threat, however, their statements implicitly relate to the threat, which may impede understanding for those who do not share the experience. Thus, listening to an interview with a patient with AIDS is an act of secondary witnessing: the audience must actively connect subjective expression and fragmentary narration to traumatic context.

In the material of the Face of AIDS film archive one can perceive how several witness roles are undertaken simultaneously. When interviewed, patients with AIDS speak as victims, eyewitnesses, and activists at the same time. What the patient is not able to express is acknowledged by the co-present audience, interviewer, cameraman, doctors, and friends via secondary witnessing. At the same time, the audience are eyewitnesses of the death of a patient, friend, or partner, and so trauma negatively affects not only the coherence of the patient's narration but that of the mediation.

Representing HIV and AIDS

Representations of HIV and AIDS in film and television can, roughly speaking, be divided into two categories: on the one hand, mainstream films, fictional melodramas, and documentaries, and, on the other, autobiographical film essays and self-reflective documentaries produced in the context of HIV and queer activism.

In the films of the first category, individuals living with HIV represent a cultural "otherness" which in earlier works that focus on HIV and AIDS "is similar in identifiable ways of otherness in other kinds of movies" (Hart 2000: 16). In melodramas, for instance, HIV and AIDS are a means of depicting family values and a traditional social structure: "Most infected individuals in AIDS movies", Hart argues, "typically die and [are] frequently members of stigmatized social groups" (Hart, 2000: 30). These stories may be based on true and authentic cases, but the deceased are portrayed from an exterior perspective wherein social norms are constructed and maintained.

Alternative videomaking counters and alters mainstream media. Alexandra Juhasz examines documentaries that offer an "alternative representational production, involving the creation of images from within the community of individuals living with and/or dying from AIDS" (Juhasz 1995 206–207). Kylo-Patrick Hart stresses the fact that the testimonial dimension is crucial in these films: "It is precisely because the images depicted in these documentaries are so intimately tied to the personal experience and interpretations of the individuals choosing to capture them that they appear to lay claim to a wider truth about HIV/AIDS" (Hart 2000: 146–147). The testimonial acts of these personal stories are further emphasised by Hallas, who argues that the personal act of witnessing in alternative queer video art enables the production of not only authentic testimonies of experiences with HIV and AIDS but also a critical perspective on the representation of the epidemic in mainstream media (2009). However, these critical perspectives and alternative testimonies only circulate within queer and HIV activist circles, and what these narratives bear witness to is not always clear to an audience that does not share the experience.

Hildebrand's early documentary films and footage are to some extent shaped by the conventions of portraying the sick body, death, homosexuality, and family norms. The exposure of patients' thin, weak bodies is combined with expert interviews, wherein doctors and scientists explain the symptoms from what is presented as an objective perspective. This combination is similar to the documentaries and TV reports that were produced during the early phase of HIV and AIDS, where, to a certain degree, the story is one of AIDS patients who are positioned as "other" to an outside viewer who is not part of the HIV activist movement.

The unedited footage in the archive, however, constitutes a different and alternative voice. Hildebrand did not have to adapt his mode of documentation to the tastes of a broad television audience and television production conventions. The first viewers of the films were audiences at HIV conferences: members of the HIV and AIDS communities who were personally engaged with and possessed knowledge of the conditions of the disease. In addition – and perhaps more importantly – the idea of creating an archive for future users or spectators had occurred to Hildebrand from the beginning (Hildebrand in this anthology). Whereas leftover footage usually is generally deselected and not intended to be seen by audiences, the leftover footage in the Face of AIDS film archive must be interpreted differently: This footage was shot to be stored, archived, and viewed by audiences in an imagined future.

In addition, Hildebrand's long engagement with HIV and AIDS connects narratives and perspectives, and establishes him as eyewitness and contemporary witness and activist. The archive provides insights into the subjective perceptions and experiences of the many people involved, and so taken together the narratives bear witness to the epidemic as an unfolding process that is reconsidered and reassessed multiple times.

AIDS has been witnessed in various forms by eyewitnesses, experts, contemporary witnesses, activists, and survivors, and some of these roles may also unite in certain people (see e.g. Cameron 2005). It has been noted that testimonial writing relating to HIV and AIDS consciously challenges strategies of othering that are designed to keep the disease at a distance (Brophy 2004). Roger

Hallas asserts that subjective narratives in alternative queer video art bear witness to the experience of HIV and AIDS (Hallas 2009).

The archive provides a space of coherence in which these different approaches meet but does not establish an overarching narrative. The archive constitutes a patchwork of stories that often contradict one another and provide alternative perspectives. Here, then, traditional forms of witnessing meet intensely subjective narratives that do not necessarily explain what they bear witness to. In the following, we intend to show how in the archive's space of coherence both mainstream narrative approaches and subjective testimonies can be seen to change over time and shed light on each other within the archive's space of coherence.

Lyle Taylor in the archive

As Hildebrand's first encounter with an individual dying from AIDS, the interview with Lyle Taylor was a pivotal moment in his documenting of the epidemic. The interview made Hildebrand's engagement more personal, which was reinforced by the fact that Taylor passed away only ten hours after the interview. According to Hildebrand's own statement in later documentaries and interviews conducted as part of the establishing of the archive, Taylor helped him to conquer his own fear of approaching patients with AIDS and assisted him in understanding that he could not document HIV and AIDS neutrally and from a distance but had to personally engage as an activist.

The interview with Taylor is included in many films, from the early documentaries *Crossover – The Global Impact of AIDS* (1988) and *AIDS – From Panic to Silence* (1998) to the later, more retrospective films *From Stigma to Hope – A Report from the Frontline of AIDS* (2011) and *Transmissions – A Journey from AIDS to HIV* (2014). There are crucial differences between the documentaries, and even more between the original interview and the documentaries. The trajectory of this interview, and how its testimony changes in relation to the changing narratives of the documentaries, is traced through each work in the following discussion.

The raw footage of the interview is over thirty minutes long, of which only a few are included in the films. In the original footage, the camera pans in and out between facial close-ups and full-frame images that show the body. As in many portraits of AIDS patients of the 1980s, images of sick bodies are part of documenting the epidemic. Hildebrand's hesitating, tentative questions regarding how Taylor's life has been changed by the diagnosis and how he experiences the related physical and psychological changes are heard off-screen. Taylor's answers are long and seemingly digressive; he avoids direct explanations and straightforward descriptions relating to the questions, and instead presents effects and causes that are seemingly far from the disease itself.

Taylor's doctor, John Dwyer, was interviewed on the same occasion. In a ten-minute piece of footage the doctor enters the room and, talking to the camera at Taylor's bedside, explains the physical state of his patient. A retrospective

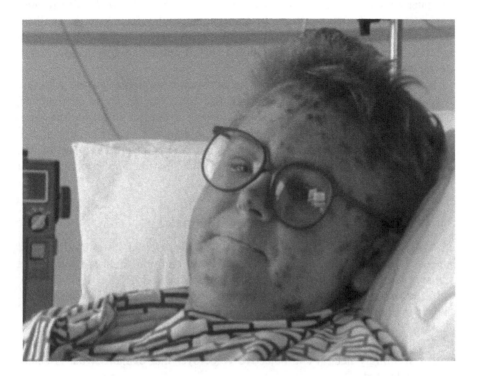

Figure 2.1 Lyle Taylor.
Source: Archive ID 1988_23.

interview conducted with Dwyer over twenty years later for the film *Trans-missions*, as well as an interview with Hildebrand himself focusing on his role as a contemporary witness, can be found on the archive's website.

Each documentary remediates essentially the same quotations from the ori-ginal interviews, but in each they relate to a different historical context and doc-umentary narrative. Although the verbal testimony remains the same, what the words bear witness to changes from film to film.

The differences between the two earliest documentaries – *Crossover* and *From Panic to Silence* – and the two most recent – *From Stigma to Hope* and *Transmissions* – are particularly striking. These are due to the fact that the story of HIV and AIDS was told differently in the 1980s and 1990s as compared to the 2010s. It is also due to Hildebrand's changed approach. The recent films are more subjective, foregrounding the testimonial dimension and Hildebrand's position as a contemporary witness to a greater extent. Here, the filmmaker's personal testimony frames the story and interacts with the testimonies of the interviewed patients, doctors, and relatives.

Within Bill Nichols's categorisation of documentary film modes, the two early films can be considered to be *expository*, while the more recent ones lie at the intersection of *participatory* and *performative* (Nichols 2017). The former construct a specific argument for the audience, and interviews function as illustrations. The perceptions and experiences of eyewitnesses, experts, and patients are intended to establish the credibility of the authoritative voice-over that develops the argument.

In the later films the interviewees collaborated to a greater degree with the filmmaker, and the films foreground the subjective experience of contemporary witnesses. Although essentially the same footage is used in all of the films, the differing approaches – from argumentative filmmaking to testimonial – afford Lyle Taylor a different status. In the early films he is an *example*, part of the evidence that is presented for the argument; in the later films he is foregrounded as a *person* with his own testimony.

Early documentaries: argumentative filmmaking

In *Crossover* and *From Panic to Silence* Taylor's verbal testimony and the image of his body serve as evidence to his fatal condition. Both are part of the films' construction of a narrative that argues that HIV and AIDS will spread globally, beyond the identified at-risk groups. *Crossover* argues that HIV and AIDS endanger all and that the condition will spread throughout the population. *From Panic to Silence* explores the dangers of not directly addressing the threat posed by HIV and AIDS. These earlier films are traditional expository documentaries, with a seemingly neutral and objective voice-over that explains what is being shown and heard.

Taylor is present in two parts of *Crossover*, while *From Panic to Silence* only includes one scene. In the part that occurs in both films, Taylor utters one phrase: "It started in the homosexual community, but it is not a homosexual disease". This utterance is not especially representative of his discourse in general – in which gay identity or sexuality is rarely foregrounded explicitly – and investigating the unedited footage reveals that this is the only point at which Taylor speaks of the homosexual community as "we", in opposition to the heterosexual community. Outside of this instance, the Western world or even humanity are "we". In relation to his verbal testimony regarding the possible future spread of HIV to heterosexuals, his body serves as evidence not only to what has happened but to what is threatened to happen in the future.

Taylor is first introduced with a medium shot of his emaciated body, covered with blue and black marks indicative of the skin cancer Kaposi's sarcoma. The neutral voice-over states that "this is a young man in his thirties", combining emotional effect and the weak and seemingly old body of the footage. The next sequence presents Doctor Dwyer in the role of expert witness, explaining the patient's physical condition to the camera. He states that his patient is dying and that they have interrupted the treatment, and testifies to Taylor's courage and acknowledges his activist attitude as "inspiring".

In this scene, the doctor's expert testimony on Taylor's condition primarily serves as evidence to the threat of AIDS. While the doctor explains the symptoms, however, Taylor's thin leg is visible in the foreground. This framing gives an ambiguity of perspective: on the one hand, the sequence is shot as a classical interview wherein the interviewee addresses the interviewer. On the other, the point of view of the camera leads to a different act of witnessing; the camera not only documents the doctor's words but mediates them from a perspective assuming Taylor's own point of view.

In the second segment, only seen in *Crossover*, Taylor explains that, against all odds, he is still alive: "I can't find the switch, to switch life off", he says with a smile. The "I am still alive" statement is the core of early HIV testimonies. At this early stage of the epidemic, most of those patients interviewed were dying. Their testimonies draw attention to the simple fact that they are "still alive". Their witnessing does not primarily say "I will soon die" but "I live now", and so makes the present moment particularly significant. Taylor's metaphor – "I can't find the switch, to switch life off" – is even more striking as he flips his index finger upwards as if to flip a switch *on*. After this statement, the voice-over explains that Lyle died the same day, retrospectively giving the inability to "switch life off" a different meaning.

Later documentaries: Taylor in retrospect and the filmmaker's testimony

In the two films from the 2010s, *From Stigma to Hope* and *Transmissions*, the archival dimension of Taylor's testimony are reinforced. To a certain extent, the subjective experience itself frames the narrative. Both films begin with the personal testimony of Hildebrand, reflecting on his journey with the Face of AIDS project. Unlike in the earlier films Hildebrand's voice (and thus his Swedish accent) is heard in the voice-over, as he looks back on the thirty years of the Face of AIDS project and explains how it has shaped him as a filmmaker and his engagement with HIV issues. In his reflections as a contemporary witness, he accords the encounter with Taylor a crucial role: in his words, it made him understand that he had to be not only a documenting filmmaker but a personally engaged "activist". The personal, auto-reflexive documentary frame of the later films also changes the interviews and testimonies of the patients, activists, and scientists, as the foregrounding of the filmmaker's personal engagement place greater focus on the dialogues and exchanges of experiences.

The same clips from the raw footage as described above are used in these two later films. There are however, minor but significant changes. Hildebrand's very first questions to Taylor are included, and we hear his off-screen voice posing the question: "Can you tell me your name?" After Taylor's answer, Hildebrand asks him to describe the experience of dying of AIDS. The presence of the filmmaker's voice at the beginning of the interview forms a bridge between the testimony of the filmmaker and that of Taylor. The latter is not, as in the earlier films, a piece of evidence to prove the overall argument of the film; rather, it is one voice among others, and each voice and statement bears witness to a personal, subjective experience.

The last film, *Transmissions*, is more explicitly archival and to a greater extent testimonial than the earlier *From Stigma to Hope*. The film is retrospective; Hildebrand returns to people he has met and interviewed in the past, shows them the early film footage, and interviews them again. This retrospective take on the film material not only highlights the differences between the perception of HIV and AIDS in the 1980s/1990s and today but reinforces the subjective experiences of the interviewees as contemporary witnesses.

In addition to the footage of Taylor and his doctor from the 1980s, *Transmissions* shows Taylor's doctor viewing this footage and Dwyer's reflections on his memories of Taylor and the original interview. He explains that, seated beside Taylor just hours before his death, he felt more like a comforting friend or psychologist than a treating doctor. In his memory, the words spoken in that moment were less explanation of the symptoms and effects of a virus than a way of addressing Taylor at this difficult time.

These reflections on the past, given in the present, change the perspective on the ten-minute interview with the doctor. In the earlier documentaries, the excerpts chosen provide "objective" explanations of the patient's physical state. In this later film, the doctor acts as contemporary witness. He expresses his personal experience of being close to a dying person and formulates the difficulty inherent in his conflicting roles as doctor, expert, friend, and eyewitness.

All four films that feature the footage of Taylor balance testimonial subjectivity and the filmmaker's argument regarding HIV and AIDS. The testimonial dimension increases in the more recent films. The subjective testimony takes an even more central role in the archive when the latter is considered as a media

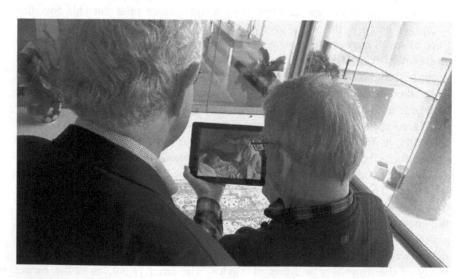

Figure 2.2 Staffan Hildebrand and John Dwyer watching the interview with Lyle Taylor from 1988. *Transmissions*.

Source: Hildebrand, 2014.

interface. Here, the raw footage of the interviews is accessible, and appended to each is a written comment and sometimes even a filmed interview in which the filmmaker reflects on the circumstances in which that particular piece of footage was shot. In the case of the Taylor interview, Hildebrand's comments on the archive's webpage add an even more intimately personal dimension to the story than that found in the later, retrospective films. Here, he describes his insecurities and fears of encountering a dying patient, and expresses guilt in relation to the fact that Taylor's death only hours after the interview may have been due to the strain that the interview situation placed on him. On Dwyer's advice, Hildebrand returned to the patient after the interview to say goodbye and shake his hand before leaving, on the basis that physical contact with an individual infected by the virus was, according to the doctor, necessary in order to truly document AIDS. This testimony relating to what happened before and after the interview becomes a frame of interpretation that facilitates an understanding of the films and film extracts featuring Taylor.

The footage: presence and subjectivity

The original footage of the interview does not have the same explicitly testimonial character as the excerpts used in the documentaries. At first glance, Taylor's verbal testimony appears to be strangely disconnected from his condition.

Although Hildebrand explicitly asks about the experience of living with HIV and dying of AIDS, Taylor's answers appear unrelated to these questions; he extensively describes the positive effects of his diagnosis and his discovery of philosophy, difficulties in starting a business, and relationship problems, and stresses the need for societal change. Nevertheless, the dark spots of Kaposi's sarcoma and his emaciated body constantly remind the viewer of his fatal condition, constantly bearing witness to the presence of AIDS. There is thus no need to verbalise what the audience can witness with their own eyes. His physical condition visibly vouches for the fact that everything said and seen expresses, in some way, the experience of HIV and AIDS. However, for anyone who does not share his experience, it is difficult to understand exactly *how* his words connect with his condition. What does this interview bear witness to, and how might it expand a viewer's understanding of AIDS?

The audience might expect a subjective expression of the lethal threat of AIDS from the testifying patient. However, Taylor largely avoids addressing the experience of AIDS verbally. Instead, what is verbally expressed becomes comprehensible *in relation to* the experience of AIDS as a lethal threat. We do not find a comprehensive narration of the experience of trauma; rather, we meet narratives that stem from experiencing a lethal threat and pain, and that can be seen as a *response* to trauma by stressing the presence of Lyle Taylor as a person.

The footage also reveals simultaneous and conflicting witness roles. Watching the interview, we both witness a victimised body and encounter a person still involved, refusing to be reduced to a victimised other. Taylor himself does not explicitly connect these two contradictory aspects of witnessing, however, as this has to be undertaken by the audience as an act of secondary witnessing.

When Taylor speaks about his condition, he uses several formulations that likely are intended to maintain a mental distance: understatements ("a bit of a shock") and modifiers ("fairly difficult"). He quickly sums up the outbreak of AIDS with a common metaphor ("all hell's broken loose"), which gains testimonial impact owing to the long silence that follows. Throughout the interview, pauses and silences, ruptures and sudden changes of topic perhaps serve as indexical signs of pain, emotion, and struggle that are not verbally expressed.

Even an apparently digressive answer may bear witness to the extremity of the situation: When Hildebrand directly asks "How close are you to being dead [*sic*]?", Taylor's answer paradoxically frames death as something that he has already repeatedly survived ("I was supposed to be dead two weeks ago"; "this morning I really thought I was dying"). This self-confident acceptance, however, is repeatedly interrupted by exclamations such as "you see, I don't know what normal is!", expressing the unprecedented, troubling character of his situation. Subjectivity, confidence, and resistance on the one hand and ongoing struggle on the other merge into one another.

Taylor focuses on the positive effects of his diagnosis, as "increased leisure" allowed him to discover literature and philosophy. His positive evaluation of a devastating situation clashes with the audience's external apprehension, but as a *response* to lethal threat, Taylor's statements bear witness to his focus on the present moment and the positive attitude and energy that the doctor testifies to.

Most confusingly to an outside viewer, Taylor describes his former, materialist lifestyle in sharp contrast to his spiritually and intellectually more rewarding one post-diagnosis. He employs a narrative pattern that resembles a religious testimonial – a narrative of conversion, centring on an experience of redemption – that seriously challenges the views of the audience, as few would term an HIV infection "redemptory". The use of this pattern could be seen as a response to a family background that Taylor describes as "fundamentalist Christian", and can be understood as an attempt to cope with traumatic challenges by applying familiar narrative patterns. However, as this pattern is used to cope with a condition that fundamentalist morals would condemn, it is simultaneously a queer and subversive act of appropriation.

The focus on the present is itself a response to trauma, and this focus pervades the interview. Taylor's personal approach to the situation expresses his appreciation of the present situation in a way that once again challenges the views of the audience, describing his stay in the palliative care facility as "like holiday" and taking clear enjoyment in telling the story of how he "attended his own wake" two weeks before.

Taylor also stresses the everyday, the normal, dwelling more on relationship- and business-related troubles than his exceptional and threatening condition. Indeed, he applies the word "trauma" to these experiences, and *not* to his lethal condition. Taylor thus presents himself as a subject that is still involved in life, insisting on his right to be caught up in "normal" troubles and not be

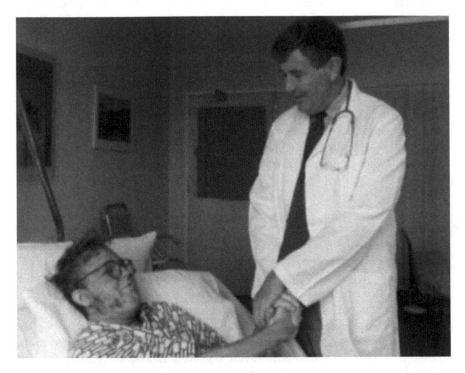

Figure 2.3 Lyle Taylor and John Dwyer shaking hands.
Source: Archive ID 1988_25.

overwhelmed by trauma. He also maintains involvement in the future, stressing the need for change in society. Taylor thus maintains subjectivity and speaks as an accepted part of society, rather than as a victimised other. Throughout the interview, Taylor presents himself as being – and remaining – involved in both the present and the future, expressing subjectivity and agency in response and resistance to the lethal threat of AIDS.

In addition, the ten minutes of footage featuring the interview with Dwyer reveals a surprising complexity. The footage starts with the call "action" and the doctor entering the room. These signs of staging do not simply produce images and statements necessary for the purposes of documentaries, however, as they may also contribute to creating meaningful, significant moments (Lanzmann 2000: 109). After the initial handshake, evidencing the fact that AIDS is not transmitted through skin-on-skin contact, the doctor sits down at Taylor's bedside and speaks with him, while simultaneously explaining Taylor's physical condition to the audience. When Hildebrand directly asks the doctor for an explicit summary of Taylor's condition, the doctor has to turn to him and the camera. Here, Taylor is excluded from the conversation, and his sick body comes more into focus.

However, this problematic shift is negotiated in several ways. First, Dwyer starts by acknowledging Taylor as an inspiring personality. Second, immediately after the summary of Taylor's devastating physical condition, Taylor himself stresses the present moment by remarking off-screen that "I just don't die". Third, the unconventional camera angle – shot from a perspective close to Taylor's own – may be an act of secondary witnessing, in that it adopts Taylor's perspective instead of showing him as a sick, othered body.

Within the documentaries, the doctor's summarising statement on Taylor's condition appears to be a conventional, expert one. The footage reveals an intricate situation wherein the need for verbalised knowledge has to be balanced and negotiated, where the audience acts as secondary witnesses.

Conclusion

In this chapter, footage of the interview with Lyle Taylor has been examined and its trajectory in the Face of AIDS film archive traced. This heterogeneous material was approached from the perspective of witnessing and testimony.

The same interview footage appears in many of the archive's documentaries. However, different overarching narratives and editing approaches affect and change the testimony of the same words and scenes.

The raw footage contains a complexity that cannot be conveyed within the frame of a documentary, as a number of narratives appear to be unrelated to the questions. It has been shown how Taylor's answers express subjectivity, agency, and social involvement. The interview can thus be seen as a subjective *response* to the experience of AIDS and the threat of being reduced to a sick, othered body.

The relationship between testimonial word and presence, body, and context can be used to clarify how the pieces of footage relate to the documentaries that they were used in, and can also assist in understanding the footage of the interview in relation to Taylor's experience of HIV and AIDS, rather than as a verbal expression of experience.

The relational approach of witnessing thus highlights the potential of the archive. In this context, the overarching narratives of edited documentaries do not tell *the* story of HIV and AIDS but constitute attempts to formulate a narrative at certain points in time and from certain perspectives. The archive also shows how the trauma of HIV and AIDS fractures the speech act of witnessing and gives rise to simultaneous and sometimes conflicting witness roles. At the same time, the archive offers a frame of understanding whenever the subjectivity of a testimony challenges our external knowledge by presenting the unexpected.

The archive engages its audience and users in the process of witnessing. The array of different perspectives and experiences that change over time presents the challenge of mediating, and any user of the archive must acknowledge these difficulties and fractures when acting as a secondary witness. The archive, with its many voices and personal testimonies, has the potential to become an interactive site where educators and activists with new perspectives and different stories may contribute to existing testimonies.

References

Assmann, Aleida (2007). "Vier Grundtypen von Zeugenschaft", in M. Elm and G. Kößler (eds), *Zeugenschaft des Holocaust: Zwischen Trauma, Tradierung und Ermittlung*, pp. 33–51. Frankfurt/Main and New York: Campus.

Baer, Ulrich, ed. (2000). *Niemand zeugt für den Zeugen: Erinnerungskultur und historische Verantwortung nach der Shoah*. Frankfurt/Main: Suhrkamp.

Brophy, Sarah (2004). *Witnessing AIDS: Writing, Testimony and the Work of Mourning*. Toronto: University of Toronto Press.

Cameron, Edwin (2005). *Witness to AIDS*. London: I.B. Taurus.

Elm, M. and G. Kößler, eds (2007). *Zeugenschaft des Holocaust: Zwischen Trauma, Tradierung und Ermittlung*. Frankfurt/Main and New York: Campus.

Engdahl, Horace (2002). "Philomena's Tongue", in H. Engdahl (ed.), *Witness Literature: Proceedings of the Nobel Centennial Symposium*, pp. 3–14. River Edge, NJ, London, Singapore and Hong Kong: World Scientific.

Englund, Peter (2002). "The Bedazzled Gaze", in H. Engdahl (ed.), *Witness Literature: Proceedings of the Nobel Centennial Symposium*, pp. 45–56. River Edge, NJ, London, Singapore and Hong Kong: World Scientific.

Hallas, Roger (2009). *Reframing Bodies: AIDS, Bearing Witness, and the Queer Moving Image*. Durham, NC: Duke University Press.

Hart, Kylo-Patrick R. (2000). *The AIDS Movie: Representing a Pandemic in Film and Television*. New York: Haworth.

Hartman, Geoffrey (2000). "Intellektuelle Zeugenschaft und die Shoah", in Ulrich Baer (ed.), *Niemand zeugt für den Zeugen: Erinnerungskultur nach der Shoah*, pp. 35–52. Frankfurt am Main: Suhrkamp.

Juhasz, Alexandra (1995). *AIDS TV: Identity, Community, and Alternative Video*. Durham, NC: Duke University Press.

Krämer, Sybille (2015). *Medium, Messenger, Transmission. An Approach to Media Philosophy*. Amsterdam: Amsterdam University Press.

Lanzmann, Claude (2000). "Der Ort und das Wort", in Ulrich Baer (ed.), *Niemand zeugt für den Zeugen: Erinnerungskultur und historische Verantwortung nach der Shoah*, pp. 101–118. Frankfurt/Main: Suhrkamp.

Levi, Primo (1988). *The Drowned and the Saved*. London: Abacus.

Nichols, Bill (2017). *Introduction to Documentary*. 3rd ed. Bloomington, IN: Indiana University Press.

Peters, John Durham (2001). "Witnessing". *Media Culture Society*, 23: 707–723.

Treichler, Paula A. (1999). *How to Have Theory in an Epidemic: Cultural Chronicles of AIDS*. Durham, NC: Duke University Press.

3 Voices of AIDS

The HIV virus and the shaping of a cultural memory

Cecilia Trenter

It has been more than thirty-five years since the global pandemic of HIV/AIDS began. Varieties of circumstances have changed both the state and the view of HIV/AIDS. From being a nameless epidemic spread predominantly among gay men, medical development and political mobilization have limited the disease and changed the status of the virus. Today HIV is a chronic but treatable condition. This redefinition of HIV has altered the way societies remember HIV/AIDS. The commemoration of AIDS differs from other traumas that are spatially as well as temporally limited to a certain event or process, marked by a starting point and an ending, e.g., the Holocaust or 9/11, as AIDS is a global and ongoing trauma (Harvey 2013). HIV/AIDS is a contemporary global epidemic and at the same time history. In communities where people can receive treatment, AIDS is no longer a current trauma, which allows opportunities for actors with public influence to create a distance to AIDS by staging the pandemic as a memory. Crucial for understanding the representation and memory of HIV/AIDS is the fact that there is a "before" and an "after" the introduction of antiretroviral therapy. The following questions are raised in the discourse about HIV/AIDS and memory: How should a generation of people living with HIV today relate to the memory of the AIDS epidemic and mass death? How should the memory of dying and AIDS be managed and by whom? Are stories about living with HIV a memory that can be paralleled to the memory culture of mass death from AIDS? How are actors formed among mainly activist groups and through which media will the stories be created? Central issues are how communities and individual actors position themselves in the memory process: as a subject (someone who remembers and represents); as an object (someone who is the subject of memory and represented); or as excluded from the stories? Another complexity in memorialization is inequalities. Both interpretations and representations of HIV/AIDS, irrespective of the nature of the intentions and gestures, expose sexism, poverty, homophobia and racism (Fink, Juhasz, Harvey and Ghosh 2013). This chapter discusses how the Face of AIDS film archive contributes to the memory of AIDS, first by discussing the commemoration processes of AIDS in terms of the differences between a communicative memory and a cultural memory, and second by taking a closer look at the documentaries *The Longest Journey Is the Journey Within* (2015) and *Passing on the Torch* (2012) in the Face of AIDS film archive.

Actors in the communicated memory and the cultural memory

The terms social memory, collective memory and cultural memory have been used during the last decade to explain memory processes such as the processing of a trauma. The term cultural memory arises from the sociologist Halbwachs's idea of social memory as a reaction to the beliefs about memory as racial and biological that predominated in the early 1900s. Instead, Halbwachs, among others, interpreted memory as a product mainly created by social circumstances such as class, profession, family and nation. Halbwachs distinguished between two kinds of social memory: everyday memory, communicated in order to maintain a group identity, and collective memory shared by professionals, the former defined as subjective memory and the latter as history (Halbwachs 1950; Landsberg 2004; Crownshaw 2014).

The Egyptologist Jan Assmann's ideas of cultural memory do not make any distinction between a subjective memory and an objective history. Instead, Assmann argues that the institutionalized memory, or cultural memory, is as socially affected as everyday communication but with other means and signs; the term cultural memory refers to a memory that is institutionalized into rituals and traditions, archives and museums or sites of memorials (Assmann 1995). The cultural memory is established at a distance from the historical event, and the past is mediated as a master narrative. Assmann refers to the Jewish calendar as an example of cultural memory based on figures of memory and ceremonially communicated memories. Assmann underlines that the distinction between the memory forms does not lie in the form of the medium; everyday memory is not defined by oral communication, nor is cultural memory defined by written texts (Assmann 1995). I consider it relevant to elaborate on that statement a little further by emphasizing that the differences lie in the ways in which the cultural memory manifests authority and impact in public; that is, a film, novel, artefact or ritual does not turn into a cultural memory unless it attains a certain status of cultural heritage or a position as an official social memory. I define the Swedish author Jonas Gardell's trilogy *Don't Ever Wipe Tears without Gloves* (2012–2013) as an example of cultural memory, as well as the Face of AIDS film archive, although the first is a novel and the latter an archive; they are both salient public producers of memory.

Everyday memory, communicative memory, is characterized by diversity in the interpretations of history, by pluralism that offers different purposes of communication and instability. In other words, it is polyphonic and multidialogical, and does not close the door between the present and past but discusses the present as an ongoing part of the past. I consider the novel *And the Band Played On: Politics, People, and the Aids Epidemic* – written by the American journalist and author Randy Shilts in 1987 and adapted for television through an HBO series in 1993, which was published before the antiretroviral medication breakthrough – as a prominent and important voice in the communicative memory. The plot covers the first years of the epidemic and starts with the illness of the

Danish doctor Grethe Rask, at that time the first known diagnosed patient, who became ill in Zaire and died of a rare pneumonia in 1977. Shilts ends the book with the officially announced death by AIDS of the actor Rock Hudson in 1985. The narrative interweaves stories from a gallery of dramatis personae, picked from different milieus that highlight political struggles, academic fights and the lack of governmental effectiveness. His work has since been integrated into the cultural memory since the drama-documentary has been evaluated as an important milestone in the memory of AIDS, and has become an important source to the history of AIDS (McKay 2014). Since Shilts's death – he died from AIDS-related complications in 1994 – he has been important in the shaping of a cultural memory in the U.S.A., although he acted as a debater in a communicated memory context. He also published *The Mayor of Castro Street* (1982), a biography of Harvey Milk, who was the first openly homosexual elected official in California and was murdered in 1978. That novel was adapted to an Oscar-winning documentary in 1984 by Rob Ebstein and became an important building-stone in the commemoration of Harvey Milk that peaked in 2007 with Gus van Sant's double Oscar-winning film *Milk* (Villa 2010).

Another example of how a communicative memory afterwards becomes part of a master narrative within the cultural memory of AIDS is the AIDS activist and writer Larry Kramer's controversial autobiographical drama *The Normal Heart* (1984). The play that was shown off-Broadway was at first a contribution to the debate on the gay movement's view of sexuality during the first years of the AIDS epidemic. In 2011 it opened on Broadway, and was finally adapted for film in 2014, and was then presented as a way of remembering AIDS (www.hollywoodreporter.com/review/normal-heart-review-anger-history-706237).

Both Shilts's and Kramer's works differ from the memorial act of Jonas Gardell. Gardell is a prominent actor in the Swedish public sphere as a stand-up comedian and author of several autobiographical novels. Gardell's internationally acclaimed trilogy *Don't Ever Wipe Tears without Gloves* (2012–2013), which was adapted for television by Simon Kaijser in 2012, belongs to an explicit cultural memory, in that the narrative directly claims to tell the history of what happened during the 1980s in Stockholm, by means of a tribute from a distance to those who died of AIDS and suffered from stigma. *Don't Ever Wipe Tears without Gloves* also has a documentary approach to the history of HIV and AIDS, but the novel is a romantic fiction in three parts (1 *Love*, 2 *Sickness* and 3 *Death*). The story is about a couple in Stockholm during the early 1980s – Benjamin, who is a former Jehovah's Witness, and Rasmus, a young man from the countryside who moves to the capital to come out of the closet – and their friends and family. There is no doubt about the drama-documentary intention despite the fictional format; Gardell begins by emphasizing the authenticity of the story; this actually did happen in Stockholm, and elsewhere, only thirty years ago. The story of the members in "the family," the group of gay men that are portrayed one by one, is mixed with information on relevant themes such as facts about the virus, homosexuality and manhood, the media image and mediation of AIDS. The story begins at the time just before the pandemic reaches Sweden and ends thirty years later.

If Shilts's drama-documentary is a whistle-blower, focusing on the chronicles and a chronological timeline by describing the development as a psychological process of trauma shaped by denial, anger, awakening and acceptance, Gardell's testimony is a memorial with a historical dimension underlined by flashbacks and fragmented narratives that together portray the memory of the gay movement group and individuals within it.

The power to position cultural memory

An important difference between communicative and cultural memory is the position of power. The communicative memory is certainly not without hierarchies but the public is accessible to everyone, especially in times of social media. Video installations, blogs, political statements and all kinds of performances that address the memory belong to communicative memory. Professionals in prominent public positions, such as historians, journalists and teachers, however, have a monopoly to communicate and define the cultural memory; histories are united into History. The preferential right of interpretation of the past is a powerful position. The transmission from the polyphonic voices in the communicative memory is characterized not only by complexity but also by conflicts and political battles about the rights and ownership of the past, the content of the memories and what values the memories should represent. The endeavor to include AIDS in a national identity expresses an awareness about the importance of defining memory as a matter of concern for the entire nation in order to achieve health-policy action. As long as AIDS was regarded as an isolated problem associated with homosexual men, the nation would never allocate funding for research and support for people living with HIV. The claim to make the AIDS issue into a national matter is present in *Angels in America: A Gay Fantasia on National Themes* (1991, adapted to an HBO miniseries in 2003) by Toni Kushner. The social memory of AIDS contains a worldwide variety of plays that articulate the trauma of AIDS, but *Angels in America* takes a full step into a cultural memory-position by claiming the definition of an overall national identity (Savran 1997). So does Gardell in his epos. He refers to artefacts that signal the typical Swedish *folkhem* ("the people's home," as the welfare state is known in Sweden) during the 1980s, for instance the way people celebrate Christmas, by letting historical events appear in a cavalcade as a background to the main plot, evoking those days in order to create a spirit of the time which he contrasts efficiently to the story of the gay community. While Kushner's drama is fiction and fantasy, Gardell claims to tell the story of what was in fact going on in Stockholm. In that sense, Gardell's epic reminds us of Shilts, who was doing journalistic research to enlighten people about what was going on, and he used the recent past to outline the story of the nameless disease that finally acquired a name and a status.

With the power to be a witness of the past goes ethical responsibility (Booth 2006; Wiklund 2012). Conflicts of interest and positions are present within the commemoration of HIV/AIDS as well. The historian Christopher Capozzola has analyzed the politics of memory on the AIDS Memorial Quilt in San Francisco. Thousands of mourning people affected by the disease contributed to an ever-growing patchwork of 44,000 panels that visualize the memory of those who died of AIDS. The memorial signified a place for official mourning acts. Cleve Jones, the executive director of the Name Project Foundation, who initiated the protest march and the memorial site, emphasized that the manifestation was apolitical. However, the memorial symbols of the gay movement's rights to mourn were discussed in terms of nationalism and Americanism. This reworking of national identity has been criticized since AIDS is neither an American affair nor merely the trauma of the Caucasian Americans' gay movement. Care and trauma became memory politics. Capozzola answers the critics by underlining the importance of raising such question as the Name Project did, and the necessity of formulating an agenda for activism that paved the way for broader definitions and health-policy actions. The gay community was efficient and instrumental in fundraising and mobilized societies, getting AIDS on the political agenda (Capozzola 2002). Activism spread to other exposed groups who by means of memory and organization became actors on the political scene. The campaign "Women don't get AIDS they just die from it," which caused a change in the definition of AIDS-related diseases to include female-related sequelae, is an illustrative example of the connection between identity politics and resource policy (Shotwell 2014). In that sense, memory politics does serve people, although they might not be included in the act of memorialization.

The activist identity has been important in the narratives about AIDS. Witness identity is connected to the different generations of activism, discussed in terms of three waves of activities (Colvin 2014). The first wave consisted of groups such as Gay Men's Health Crisis, launched in 1982, as a reaction to what at that time was referred to as "gay cancer." Their aim was to provide palliative care to the sick and dying people and to fight homophobia and dehumanization of people living with HIV. The second wave involved political lobbyists and fundraising groups with the main purpose of putting AIDS on the health-policy agenda, for example ACT UP, which started in New York in 1987 at the Lesbian and Gay Community Services Center and was later spread to London and Paris. Taking shape after the breakthrough of antiretroviral therapy in the mid-1990s, the third wave focused on partnerships between activists in the developed and developing worlds, such as AIDS Action, created in 1994 as an organization for health and care, and by 2011 merged with the National AIDS Fund into AIDS United.

Commemorations started already during the second wave, for example, with the ACT UP Oral History Project, the invention of the red ribbon symbols (since 1991), a variety of plays (Francis 2011), of which *Angels in America* stands out in terms of international and public spread, and the Memorial Quilt in San Francisco. Cultural memory grows even stronger during the third wave, in which Gardell's epic drama belongs. There are several audiovisual documentaries of the memory of HIV/AIDS, from video installations to documentations of events, people and phenomena related to HIV/AIDS in order to enlighten and sometimes educate the audience. AIDS activist and filmmaker Alexandra Juhasz believes that the primary purpose of contemporary video installations is to testify, to grieve for the memory of the dead, while the early AIDS video installations described trauma and the current crisis (Juhasz 2010). Ryan Conrad's *Things Are Different Now* (2012) is an example of the autobiographical experimental film that pays attention to the grief of a lost generation. The "young faggot," as Conrad puts it, contemplates the feeling of loss in the fact that he will never meet all the people who have died from AIDS. There are examples of prize-winning and internationally acclaimed documentary films that handle aspects of memories, mostly about American activist history. *We Were Here* (David Weissman and Bill Weber, 2010), *Sex in an Epidemic* (Jean Carlomusto, 2010), *How to Survive a Plague* (David France, 2012) and *30 Years from Here: A Personal History of NYC & HIV/AIDS* (Josh Rozenzweig, 2013) are documentary films based on archival footage primarily from the 1980s, including interviews, demonstrations and meetings. The archival footage is interwoven with oral histories from people in the present who reflect on memories of the stigma, the fight for medical care, and their experiences. The biographical documentary film is yet another genre of mediating memory. *Vito* (Jeffrey Schwarz, 2011) is based on the biography of the prominent gay activist Vito Russo, and *Derek* (Isaac Julien, 2009) about the British writer and director Derek Jarman. These films convey intimate and close-up portraits of famous persons who both died of the complications of AIDS. It has been stressed that popular images such as *How to Survive a Plague* are all about white men's struggle for survival that, against all odds, succeeded. There is limited place in such a master narrative for women and queers of color, who are marginalized to victims and losers of the fight (Cheng 2016). *Fire in the Blood* (Dylan Mohan Gray, 2013) belongs to yet another genre. The film is a critical retrospective documentary film that exposes how Western pharmaceutical companies, with the consent of the governments, efficiently prevented low-cost antiretroviral therapy from reaching countries of the Global South, and how activism, particularly in South Africa, fought to get rid of the monopoly.

Alongside the documentary films, the institutionalization has been shaped by the annual international conferences and global networks. Cultural heritage – such as installations, plays, exhibitions, novels and films – is shaping a social memory that includes numerous voices in communicative memory processes that pave the way in parallel for a cultural memory. The commemoration of AIDS has been rapid and efficient. Assmann discusses the transformation from a communicative memory to a cultural memory in a long-term perspective (Assmann 1988). One could argue that the process is rapidly accelerated in the form that social memory takes in modern technology such as digital media (Landsberg 2004). Media documentation of HIV/AIDS is outstanding even by contemporary standards and within a range of contexts and purposes: artistic, documentary, scientific, informative journalism etc. The flow of mediated expressions creates a metanarrative that does not consider the chronology, but presents a polyphony of statements on HIV and AIDS from different times over a period of thirty-five years. The cultural objectified memory, for example documentary films, develops parallel to the communicated memory. Alterations in technologies as well as in science and medication, and the passage of time, challenge the representational history; what is HIV and AIDS when you are not dying of it, and when you are? (Fink, Juhasz, Harvey and Ghosh 2013). How does the Face of AIDS film archive reflect this complex process of memorialization?

The Face of AIDS film archive within the process of memorialization in two documentary films

The Face of AIDS film archive is a part of as well as a contributor to the cultural memory of HIV/AIDS. Its name, the Face of AIDS, had been used before in the commemoration of AIDS. The photographer Therese Frare's pictures of the dying thirty-two-year-old David Kirby, donated by his family, were published in 1990 in *Life*. Her pictures were named *The Face of AIDS* since the motif of the deathbed with the dying man and his relatives in despair visualized and humanized the victims of AIDS. The image became famous worldwide, and even used in commercials for the clothing company Benetton (http://100photos.time.com/photos/therese-frare-face-aids). The name of the archive is in its own right referential to the social memory of AIDS. Hildebrand donated the film material in 2015 to Karolinska Institutet at a time when the AIDS condition, thanks to antiretroviral therapy, had become history. The film material is organized according to the principle of using the history about HIV/AIDS in order to enlighten and educate people. Establishing an archive is in itself a memorial act. In the same spirit as the ACT UP Oral History Project, Hildebrand's donation of his documentation was an act of activism to ensure that the history of AIDS became known. The concrete identity of the archive's founder is that of the activist, and from this perspective the capacity for reconstructing the past forms the core of the archive. In the mnemohistory of AIDS, the transmission from communicated social memory to institutionalized cultural memory is not a homogeneous process. The historian's challenge consists of finding sources for the communicated historical memories, because they are reused in the transformation into a cultural memory. The Face of AIDS film archive delivers unique sources of perceptions of HIV and AIDS, formulated by scientists, doctors, journalists, sex buyers, people diagnosed with HIV, activists, anonymous people randomly picked for an interview, stigmatized groups such as homosexual men, drug dealers and sex workers, and politicians in the health and care sector. The unedited film material mediates the interviews with interruptions and retakes and thereby creates narratives characterized by repetitions and variations in a way that corresponds to Assmann's definition of a communicative memory. By viewing the raw material, we get to know more about the communicative memory prior to and parallel to the establishment of cultural memory which is represented in the documentaries. The way people relate to HIV and AIDS is an important source for the understanding of a trauma as well.

The Face of AIDS film archive has a unique position as a gathering point for the complex history of HIV since the archive contains material of both spatial and temporal breadth that bridges inequalities. By serving as a platform for social memory, the archive creates not only an overview of the thirty-five-year history process but also a mouthpiece of collective group identities for activists around the world. Hildebrand approaches the past in different ways in his films but always in a dialectic motion between the past, the present and the future, thereby dealing with the past of AIDS in a complex way. For example, in the documentary film *The Longest Journey Is the Journey Within* (2015), about the HIV activist Steve Sjöquist, who was diagnosed with HIV and was one of the first Swedish AIDS patients that was treated with antiretroviral medication, Hildebrand encounters the past through Sjöquist's memories. In *Passing on the Torch* (2012), Hildebrand uses his own memories to focus on the present situation and the new generation of activists.

The Longest Journey Is the Journey Within tells us a life story of Steve Sjöquist mediated by his memories and thoughts, reflected and visualized by Sjöquist visiting locations that represent his personal history. There are no facts about AIDS but only comments and reflections mediated by artistic concepts; the life story includes music that has meant much to him, a play about fear and sorrow in the wake of AIDS that Sjöquist watches and discusses afterwards with the actors. The film returns to quotations from Dag Hammarskjöld, one of which is the title of the documentary film, in order to illustrate Steve's life experience, which is characterized by faith, humility and hope, and thoughtful grieving for those who did not survive. No shame or guilt is exposed in the documentary films by Hildebrand as in, for example, Gardell's testimony. The guilt of being a survivor is present within the narrative in *Don't Ever Wipe Tears without Gloves*, through the character of Benjamin. Narratives of love, humanity and bravery are interwoven with portraits of victims, sacrifices, disgrace and guilt among the gay men who make up Rasmus and Benjamin's group of friends. The testimony is integrated into the story of Benjamin, who is raised as a Jehovah's Witness but expelled from the sect as well as from his biological family when he comes out as homosexual. The concluding scene portrays a middle-aged Benjamin, who has survived the plague and now takes part in the Pride parade in Stockholm twenty-five years later. He is still a witness but in another sense.

Steve Sjöquist is also a survivor and a witness, but Hildebrand arranges the life story in a way that highlights faith and hopefulness and a belief in the future. For example, in a scene where Steve visits the hospital ward at Södersjukhuset, where he spent a year in 1996, the ward is empty and preserves no signs of the sick and dying people that filled the rooms and corridors at that time. Steve remembers that the ward was slowly emptied as medicine caused the patients to survive and recover. Sjöquist ends the scene at the empty ward by telling us that the ward nowadays is a maternity ward. The connection between death and life is explicitly highlighted in the scene.

Hildebrand does not let Sjöquist tell the story about the sickness during the complication from AIDS that nearly took his life before he got treatment, but lets the doctor who was responsible for Sjöquist meet him in a warm and fond reunion, to tell him once again about the fight against time and the life-threatening

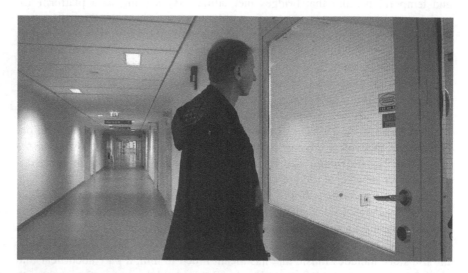

Figure 3.1 Steve outside the maternity ward. *The Longest Journey Is the Journey Within.*
Source: Hildebrand, 2015.

conditions Sjöquist was suffering from. The doctor's story reflects not only what was happening to Sjöquist but also how he himself got involved, how he thought and felt. The biographical pictures of Steve Sjöquist are created in dialectical correspondence with the doctor; Steve Sjöquist's life story is intimately connected to other people who mediate the message that Steve Sjöquist was never alone, not even when he was unconscious at Södersjukhuset.

The use of history in order to highlight not only progress but a connection between history and the present is pronounced within the documentary *Passing on the Torch* (2012), which presents the significance of activism in retrospective. Hildebrand begins by describing how he became an activist. He returns to Australia for the Pride festival in 2014 and recaps the journey in 1988 when he first met a patient dying from AIDS. Bill Bowtell, the chief of staff to the Australian minister for health 1983–1987, explains the distance between the present situation and the 1990s by saying that to young people of today the AIDS epidemic is a distant history, as distant as World War I. In addition to pointing out the good results, the documentary highlights the challenge of "passing on the torch," to ensure that the information and education about HIV and AIDS does not fall into oblivion. We do not talk about AIDS because there is efficient medication. The connection between the memory of AIDS, the nowadays-treatable HIV and behavior among the young is discussed by the activist Nic Holas as problematic and complex: how can people learn to have safe sex when AIDS is not a problem any longer?

The documentary also focuses on young people of today by delving into the situation of the actor Sebastian Robertson, who is presented as openly gay.

Robertson is also directly involved in the cultural memory of AIDS by playing in *The Death of Kings* by Adam Deusien, which was performed during the Twentieth International AIDS Conference in Melbourne in 2014. Hildebrand presents the play, which is about the AIDS epidemic in Sydney during the 1980s, and emphasizes its authenticity. "And it is based on real interviews with people that were there?" he asks, and Robertson confirms: "Yes, word for word." Scenes of the actors on stage are interwoven with an interview with one of the actual persons, the health minister's chief of staff Bill Bowtell, while Robertson is sitting next to him. Bowtell says, "It's not just my words spoken by an actor. Sebastian is bringing a great deal of himself, his understanding and his thoughts." Bowtell tells about his own experience of AIDS since his boyfriend died from it in 1987. In the next shot, Robertson is walking on an empty beach in Sydney and Hildebrand's voice-over tells us that something dramatic happened during the rehearsal of the play. In the next scene, in close-up with Robertson, Hildebrand asks if he was diagnosed with HIV, and Sebastian confirms in a single "yes." He tells his story and moves on to the stigma of HIV, which he ascribes to a lack of education.

Hildebrand returns to South Korea and Australia, which have been successful in preventing the spread of HIV. Clips from previous documentaries and interviews with activists and doctors alternate with follow-up interviews. By hovering between an earlier (historical) situation and the present, Hildebrand mediates change and progress. He deepens the insight of progress by showing shots with the interviewed activists from previous films in which they appeared.

The Face of AIDS film archive and the cultural memory of HIV/AIDS

Staffan Hildebrand's collection of 700 hours of film material represents Hildebrand as an activist. Owing to its geographical breadth (the archive reflects varied environments and about forty different countries), time duration (over thirty years) and character (sources are both edited and raw materials), the huge amount of sources is a dynamic contribution to the cultural memory of HIV/AIDS. The commemoration of HIV/AIDS is both political and complicated since the historical progress mostly reflects changes such as the medical breakthrough that changed the focus from a disease with a deadly outcome to a treatable condition. Although HIV/AIDS is a global issue, economic inequalities make the commemoration of the virus fragmented. Since the right to claim the past by defining the stories is an act of politics with consequences for the outlook on HIV/AIDS, on society and on people, the act brings a responsibility. To what extent is the cultural memory available to people? Is the purpose of the institutionalized memory transparent? What moral-didactic messages are formulated within the cultural memory? The Face of AIDS film archive presents a consciousness of pluralism that overbridges the asymmetric memorialization processes of AIDS. The archive is a platform for a transparent and hopeful narrative about the history of AIDS. It does not present *the* story and not even *one* story but polyphonically composite narratives that are filtered through a hopeful belief in the future.

References

100 Photos (n.d.). http://100photos.time.com/photos/therese-frare-face-aids, last accessed August 21, 2017.
Assmann, Jan (1995). "Collective Memory and Cultural Identity," *New German Critique*, 65(Spring–Summer): 125–133.
Booth, James W. (2006). *Communities of Memory. On Witness, Identity, and Justice.* Ithaca, NY: Cornell University Press.
Capozzola, Christopher (2002). "A Very American Epidemic: Memory Politics and Identity Politics in the AIDS Memorial Quilt, 1985–1993," *Radical History Review*, 82(Winter): 91–109.
Cheng, Jih Fey (2016). "How to Survive: Aids and Its Afterlives in Popular Media," *WSQ: Women's Studies Quarterly*, 44(1–2): 73–92.
Colvin, Christopher J. (2014). "Evidence and AIDS activism: HIV Scale-Up and the Contemporary Politics of Knowledge in Global Public Health," *Global Public Health: An International Journal for Research, Policy and Practice*, 9(1–2): 57–72.
Crownshaw, Richard (2014). "History and Memoralization," in Stefan Berger and Bill Niven (eds.), *Writing the History of Memory*. London: Bloomsbury Academic.
Fink, Marty *et al.* (2013). "Ghost Stories: An Introduction," *Jump Cut, a Review of Contemporary Media*, (Fall), www.ejumpcut.org/archive/jc55.2013/AidsHivIntroduction/index.html, last accessed May 2, 2018.
Francis, Dennis A., ed. (2011). *Acting on HIV: Using Drama to Create Possibilities for Change*. Rotterdam: Sense.
Gardell, Jonas (2012). *Torka aldrig tårar utan handskar. 1. Kärleken.* Nordstedts: Stockholm.
Gardell, Jonas (2013). *Torka aldrig tårar utan handskar. 2. Sjukdomen.* Nordstedts: Stockholm.
Gardell, Jonas (2014). *Torka aldrig tårar utan handskar. 3. Döden.* Norstedts: Stockholm.
Goodman, Tim (2014). *"The Normal Heart": TV Review*, 10:59 AM PDT 5/21, www.hollywoodreporter.com/review/normal-heart-review-anger-history-706237, last accessed August 21, 2017.
Harvey, David Oscar (2013). "Ghosts Caught in our Throat – of the Lack of Contemporary Representations of Gay/Bisexual Men and HIV," *Jump Cut, a Review of Contemporary Media*, (Fall), www.ejumpcut.org/archive/jc55.2013/AidsHivIntroduction/index.html, last accessed May 2, 2018.
Juhasz, Alexandra (2010). "AIDS Video: To *Dream* and Dance with Censor," *Jump Cut, a Review of Contemporary Media*, 52(Summer).
Kramer, Larry (2011 [1985]). *The Normal Heart*. London: Nick Hern.
Kushner, Tony (2013 [1994]). *Angels in America: A Gay Fantasia on National Themes.* New York: Theatre Communications Group.
Landsberg, Alison (2004). *Prosthetic Memory. The Transformation of American Remembrance in the Age of Mass Culture*. New York: Columbia University Press.
McKay, Richard (2014). "'Patient Zero': The Absence of a Patient's View of the Early North American AIDS Epidemic," *Bulletin of the History of Medicine* (Spring): 161–194.

Savran, David (1997). "Ambivalence, Utopia, and a Queer Sort of Materialism: How 'Angels in America' Reconstructs the Nation," *Theatre Journal*, 47(2) (May 1995): 207.
Shilts, Randy (1987). *And the Band Played on: Politics, People, and the Aids Epidemic*. New York: Penguin.
Shilts, Randy (2008 [1982]). *The Mayor of Castro Street: The Life and Times of Harvey Milk*. New York: St. Martin's Griffin.
Shotwell, Alexis (2014). "'Women Don't Get AIDS, They Just Die From It': Memory, Classification, and the Campaign to Change the Definition of AIDS," *Hypatia: A Journal of Feminism Philosophy*, 29(2) (Spring): 509–525.
Villa, Sara (2010). "Milk (2008) and The Times of Harvey Milk (1984): The Double Filmic Resurrection of the Mayor of Castro Street," *Otras Modernidades, Saggi/ Ensayos/Essais/Essays*, 3(March).
Wiklund, Martin (2012). *Historia som domstol. Historisk värdering och retorisk argumentation kring "68."* Nora: Nya Doxa.

Films and TV production

Carlomusto, Jean, *Sex in an Epidemic* (2010).
Conrad, Ryan, *Things Are Different Now* (2012).
Dylan Mohan Gray, *Fire in the Blood* (2013).
Epstein, Rob, *The Times of Harvey Milk* (1984).
Hildebrand, Staffan, *Passing on the Torch* (2012).
Hildebrand, Staffan, *Den längsta resan är resan inåt. Filmen om Steve* (2015).
Isaac, Julien, *Derek* (2009).
Kaijser, Simon, *Torka aldrig tårar utan handskar* (2012).
Nichols, Mike, *Angels in America* (2003).
France, David, *How to Survive a Plague* (2012).
Rozenzweig, Josh, *30 Years from Here: A Personal History of NYC & HIV/AIDS* (2013).
Schwarz, Jeffrey, *Vito* (2011).
van Sant, Gus, *Milk* (2008).
Weissman, David and Bill Weber, *We Were Here* (2010).

4 "A disease on top of a disease"

People with hemophilia through the Face of AIDS film archive

Daniel Normark

I'm convinced that AIDS was caused by infected blood that was used by various manufacturers of a product called factor VIII which is the medicine that hemophiliacs must take to live. To stop their bleeding. This miraculous drug started being manufactured for hemophiliacs in the mid- or late 1970s by four specific companies: Baxter Travenol, Alpha Therapeutic, Armour Pharmaceutical and Green star in Japan. And this blood is made from plasma collected from hundreds to thousands of donors. It's all pooled together this blood and in each factor VIII injection there is plasma from at least twenty thousand people because it's all pooled together and then reduced. And many of the people from where this blood was collected in the late 1970s were infected with HIV. It was collected all over the world, it was collected in South America, in the far East and especially in Africa and here from prisons and prisoners and we know that HIV was in the population of certain populations from this time on.

What is awful about all of this is that these companies knew this blood was tainted and still used it… Their excuse was a very feeble one: "that hemophiliacs were going to die anyway, this was going to give them a little longer [life]." Hemophiliacs were not living for long; the average age was in the teens before factor VIII came along. So they were given extra life so what if you have some infections from some viruses.

Gay hemophiliacs getting an infection of something with HIV in it would be infected and because gay people at that time were living enormously energetic sex-lives, everywhere especially here in America, especially here at places like Rhode Island, I believe that gay hemophiliacs are the ones that got the HIV to the gay population infected so effectively…. *It's the greed of the capitalism of these companies to put out a product that they knew was tainted that really allowed this plague to happen.*

(FoA: 2006_1, emphasis added by author)

The quote above is gay activist Larry Kramer's reaction to the question of the origins of AIDS raised by the documentary filmmaker Staffan Hildebrand. The entire interview, available in the Face of AIDS film archive, is approximately one hour long and emotionally tense. Larry Kramer expresses with resentment all his different experiences with AIDS, AIDS activism and the society at large. At the beginning of the interview he comments that the only thing he has learned during his twenty-five years of being a gay activist is "how awful people all are" (FoA:2006_1). According to what Hildebrand told me in a personal conversation, Larry Kramer was initially reluctant to participate in an interview but was persuaded by Philip Pizzo. As an author and activist who had experienced the entire story of AIDS in the U.S.A., Kramer provided an activist's perspective to most of the topics related to the U.S. AIDS history. However, in this chapter I will only unravel one of the many threads within the interview (and the archive), by focusing on the people with hemophilia and their specific role in the tragedy that we can call the history of AIDS.

People with hemophilia are a specific subset of patients. Using the accounts of hemophilia in the Face of AIDS film archive as a way to structure this chapter, I will portray their significance against a backdrop of medical history and other histories of hemophilia and HIV. Most of the headings in this chapter are quotes from interviews in the Face of AIDS film archive. For example, the title of this chapter is Philip Pizzo's description of the double tragedy of HIV and AIDS in the hemophilia community (FoA: 2006_7_04). While this double tragedy is the main focus, the variation of different historical sources also enables me to compare the similarities and differences between textual archives and audiovisual archives. I will argue that much can be gained by combining audiovisual archives with more traditional ones, without losing focus on the particular strengths of audiovisual sources.

For instance, in the above mentioned interview, Kramer acknowledges that his theory on the origin of AIDS is an interpretation of the Pulitzer Prize-winning journalist Laurie Garrett and her book *The Coming Plague* (1994). Garrett's book gives another account of the U.S. companies that sold and distributed factor VIII, namely: Baxter Travenol Laboratories, Inc., Alpha Therapeutic Corporation, Armour Pharmaceutical Co. (a division of the Revlon Cosmetics corporation) and Cutter Laboratories (Garrett 1994: 311). The book also contains many reports and documents from the CDC that confirm many of the statements made by the informants in the FoA archive.

The audiovisual media of video is something other than a written text, allowing other expressions and appeals to other senses. It is aesthetically different from a text. As Marshall McLuhan (2003) argued, the type of medium is important and the media form is part of the message, an association in itself, with particular importance. A story told through a film can appeal to emotions in different ways than a display of objects or a text can. Hence, a historical account that relies on films rather than text documents can highlight other features of a story. The interviews in the Face of AIDS film archive feel vivid and alive – something that sometimes is difficult to accomplish textually. Combining the statements in the interviews into a narrative makes one feel the experiences, excitement, fear, frustration, anger and despair that are associated with a disease such as AIDS. Here, textual archives and the Face of AIDS film archive supplement each other. Documents, reports, letters and other archival material, however, often make an account more plausible.

Larry Kramer's response unfolds several dimensions regarding hemophilia's role within the history of AIDS and the specific conditions of hemophilia that made them vulnerable to the disease. He describes the process of developing factor VIII and how fragile the system was to contamination. Kramer highlights how dependent people with hemophilia are on factor VIII – the drug really changed their life dramatically. He also explains that the production of factor VIII relied on massive collections of donated blood. Within this production process, secondary diseases caused by the treatment with factor VIII were regarded as acceptable, considering the short life expectancy of people with hemophilia. This industrial manufacturing process placed the disease, and the control of spreading it, in the hands of the companies, and subsequently in the capitalistic system where greed and profit could pave way for ignorance and neglect. Finally, arguing that people with hemophilia were infected before the gay community shifts the scope morally. It was not sex and lust that initially ignited the plague but greed. While it is important to note that the comments made by Kramer are speculations, they provide an insight into the way people born with hemophilia were affected by AIDS but also how AIDS – and the communities created in its pathway – were affected by hemophilia.

The Face of AIDS film archive – an audiovisual source

Using the archive's search engine with the MeSH terms "Hemophilia A" and "Blood transfusion," a small but manageable number of films to analyze was obtained. In total the search resulted in eighteen films, of which four were either duplicates or had insufficient sound. Hence, fourteen films remained. Of these, one film is an edited documentary and the rest are unedited footage of interviews. Because three of the unedited films were based on the same interview, my analysis is built on one edited film and eleven interviews. The film *America and AIDS – A 25 Year Perspective* was made by Hildebrand as an assignment from Dr. Antony Fauci for the twenty-fifth anniversary of the federal NIH research on HIV/AIDS. Three of the unedited interviews were, presumably, conducted when making this film, since parts of them appear in it.

Taken together, the interviews in the Face of AIDS archive resemble the various oral history projects that have focused on AIDS such as the early work at National Institutes of Health (https://history.nih.gov/NIHinownwords/index. html), the ACT UP Oral History Project (www.actuporalhistory.org/) and the HIV Story Project (http://thehivstoryproject.org/hsp/). I have regarded these interviews as my empirical material. Most of the interviews were made in the U.S., but one film was shot in Italy (1988), one in South Africa (1998) and one in Zambia (2007). The films were shot between 1988 and 2007. The interviewees were James Curran, Larry Kramer, Philip Pizzo, Harold Jaffe, Alvin Friedman-Kien, Sarah Sayifwanda, Mangalasseril G. Sarngadharan, Sten Vermund and Quarraisha Abdool Karim. All these interviewees have official standings in different ways, hence they speak as public persons. Three of the informants, who are patients or physicians in the field, were, however, made anonymous in the public part of the Face of AIDS film archive. Because of this, they will be treated anonymously in this text too. The interview with Sarah

Sayifwanda (Zambia) and Quarraisha Abdool Karim (South Africa) highlighted the role of blood banks as the main site of screening the population for HIV. As such they broadened the scope but did not add to the understanding of hemophilia and AIDS. Therefore, this chapter will focus on a U.S. history of AIDS: the discussions of the effects of hemophilia and AIDS, the cases of patients, the CDC and other actors, the reactions of communities in uproar and the governmental legislation, all refer to a U.S. setting. This approach may provide a different story than other approaches to hemophilia and AIDS that are found in academic literature, primarily based on conventional archival research (Feldman and Bayer 1999; Bovens, Hart and Peters 2001).

Methodologically, there are some challenges in trying to understand a historical process through a collection of filmed interviews. These interviews are often part of a filmmaking process, where the aim has been to tell a compelling, yet accurate, story. The aim is seldom to create complete accounts, especially for a subsidiary topic such as hemophilia. An oral history project exclusively focusing on hemophilia would create a much more nuanced narrative. However, at the same time, there is also a high degree of sincerity in the presence of issues of hemophilia within these interviews, considering that the informants talked about this topic spontaneously and not as a response to the interviewer's questions.

Focusing on interviews as the basis for an historical account, available in the Face of AIDS film archive, does not provide the same level of complexity that textual sources can provide. The descriptions in the interviews are at times sketchy since they are associations of what one remembers, and one informant, Sven Vermund, even merged Ricky Ray and Ryan White into a single individual with multiple experiences (I will return to describing who Ray and White were later in the chapter). In this chapter I will supplement the accounts made by the informants in the Face of AIDS film archive with secondary literature on AIDS and hemophilia as well as conventional archive material from a hemophilia physician (the personal archive of Margareta Blombäck; for a description see Blombäck, M. 2011a; 2011b).

I will start by describing hemophilia and how AIDS affected the hemophilia community. From there I will describe how AIDS, the understanding of the disease but also society's reaction to it, were affected by hemophilia. The understanding of AIDS changed through the discovery of AIDS among people with hemophilia. It changed the understanding of the disease, the communities of both AIDS activists, gay activists and people with hemophilia and it is the mutual transitions that took place in the different communities that I want to draw the readers' attention to.

The story of hemophilia

Hemophilia is a hereditary disease that some might associate with the "blue" blood of royal families, such as the descendants of Queen Victoria of England (1819–1901). Even though many regard it as one disease (and my text treats it as one) it is an umbrella phrase for several diseases that all have in common deficiencies in the human blood that manifest in difficulties for the blood to coagulate.

During the twentieth century the understanding of hemophilia increased as the insights into the complexity of blood grew (see for example Stormorken 2005; Blombäck, B. 2007; Berner 2012). Hemophilia is caused by suppression of one or several factors within the blood. Most common is hemophilia A, where the blood lacks factor VIII, initially called antihemophilic globulin, which is a large, instable molecule in the blood (in very low concentrations) that is also connected to other molecules (factors) in the blood that work somewhat differently, such as the von Willerbrand factor. People with hemophilia that are born without the von Willerbrand factor have the von Willerbrand disease, whereas those with hemophilia B are missing the coagulation factor IX, or the plasma thromboplastin component. These are a few of a series of molecules in the blood that together work to make the blood coagulate at the right time and place, and the theories of how that works have varied considerably during the twentieth century (as well as the nomenclature) (Stormorken 2005). Blood is a sensitive substance in which a series of different molecules and chemical substances are expected to act and react in the right place at the right time. For people with hemophilia this does not work and instead they bleed – to death. Prior to the development of substances with factor VIII, people with hemophilia risked their lives when scraping a knee, biting the tongue or during menstruation; even losing a tooth could be lethal. Hence, the way Larry Kramer described the life for people with hemophilia was accurate, a limited, painful life, highly over-protected, with short life expectancies (few grew older than twenty-five, with an average age of 11.2 years; see Garrett 1994) and no future. At first the only treatments available were regular transfusions of blood, and sterilization of relatives was also recommended (Sköld 1944). In the first half of the twentieth century many people with hemophilia were surveyed (such as in 1944 in Sweden, identifying sixty families). In Sweden, this process was conducted in close proximity to the implementation and expansion of blood banks (Berner 2012). One could argue that this created a bond, a relationship of trust between physicians specializing on hemophilia, blood banks and the family-centered hemophilia communities.

When factor VIII became available as a treatment, life shifted dramatically for the better for the entire community.[1] By fractioning out factor VIII and factor IX from human blood, a concentration of the substance could be procured that enabled the blood to coagulate when it should. Administering the drug preemptively (i.e., even though the patient is not currently bleeding) meant that an "almost" normal life could be within reach for the patient.

"Suddenly the whole picture looked much different"

Like many narratives in the history of AIDS, the story about hemophilia is a tragedy but also a game changer, a new understanding of the disease, that in turn led to an improved accuracy on what AIDS presumably could be. The AIDS story in U.S.A. usually begins with the first reported cases in 1981, in Los Angeles, San Francisco and New York. The case reports from these cities, both at these sites and at the Centers for Disease Control and Prevention (CDC), launched an investigation trying to figure out what it was that they had discovered: what the symptoms that could be related to the disease were and what could possibly cause it (FoA: 2006_9_01; FoA: 2006_9_02; FoA: 2006_10; FoA: 2007_40; FoA: 2007_41; also Garrett 1994). According to Harold Jaffe and James Curran, CDC quickly put together groups of investigators that interviewed patients in the major American cities in order to identify the possible reason why these young men were infected. The common denominator for these first patients was that they were young, highly sexually active gay men. Soon injecting drug users were included into the mapping of the disease. Being handled by the section of CDC that focused on sexually transmitted diseases (STDs), AIDS quickly became understood as a lifestyle infection. All the data indicated that this was something new, and that it was something that affected the gay population.

Medical historian William Bynum argues that (Western) medicine can be divided into five different kinds of medicine, five different ways of approaching and understanding a disease. These different kinds of medicine have dominated different periods of time but have also coexisted (Bynum, 2008). They are: bedside medicine, library medicine, hospital medicine, social medicine and laboratory medicine. Only the last three categories are, however, relevant in this chapter. The approach to understanding AIDS, at the time it was discovered, by describing the patients' behavior and the similarities between the patients resembles the logic that Bynum described as hospital medicine. Hospital medicine, according to Bynum, was developed in major cities such as London and Paris (Hotel Dieu) in the beginning of the nineteenth century as physicians became more skilled in comparing corpses pathologically with symptoms of patients. The collection of patients and the comparison of symptoms enabled the doctors to conclude that the patients were suffering from the same disease. Even though they knew very little about how the disease worked, the studies stabilized a coherent picture of what it was. In the case of AIDS, the initial observations made by the physicians in the cities and CDC resembled this practice.

In addition, the investigators at CDC specializing on sexually transmitted diseases, understood that it could also be a kind of social medicine (what Bynum refers to as the observation of communities in order to prevent diseases), mapping the habits, whereabouts and behavior of the patients. As Sten Vermund argues, they pointed toward the "early observation of the behavioral origin of risk" (FoA: 2003_7_02) – the infected men were gay and more sexually active than their noninfected equivalent. Hence, many researchers and physicians assumed that the infections would stay within this lifestyle group.

Consequently, there was skepticism and disbelief when reports came about patients with hemophilia who also displayed the same symptoms as AIDS patients. These patients did not fit the categories of previous patients. In the words of Harold Jaffe:

In the mid-fall in 1982 suddenly we started learning about other people with AIDS, we heard about a baby in San Francisco with a disease that seemed very similar, we had heard about one or two people with hemophilia and then we learned about cases in young infants in New Jersey in New York and in San Francisco, *so suddenly the whole picture looked much different.* There must be other routes of transmission besides gay sex.

(FoA: 2007_40, emphasis by author)

AIDS in people with hemophilia was "one of the *out of lifestyle* infections" (FoA: 2003_9_02, emphasis by author), i.e., that the lifestyle could not be blamed as a cause of the infection or, as James Curran commented, with people with hemophilia there was "no known behavioral risk factor" (FoA: 2006_9_01). Hence there had to be another explanation for their infections. The way hemophilia, tragically, was incorporated into the story about AIDS was one of a shifting direction of the investigation – as a step toward clearer comprehension – but at the cost of several lives.

Among the physicians and investigators, including the researchers at Advanced Bioscience Laboratories, this led to the reduction of possible models for understanding the disease – getting closer to the understanding of the virus before they knew it was a virus (FoA: 2003_9_02). At that time, CDC were struggling with different hypotheses for how the disease worked, drawing from their knowledge on sexually transmitted diseases. They were wondering if AIDS behaved like gonorrhea or like hepatitis (FoA: 2007_40).

As Harold Jaffe points out, people with hemophilia suffering from AIDS drew the attention toward hepatitis B, a disease that also became common among people with hemophilia as a side effect of the factor VIII drugs developed throughout the second part of the twentieth century. Thus they could continue investigating AIDS by searching for patterns resembling hepatitis, even though that was a more complicated model (which James Curran was an expert on). As Curran described:

The other hypothesis of lifestyle, drugs or other things just could not fit the hypothesis that persons of hemophilia would have the same condition that gay men and drug users had.

(FoA: 2006_10)

According to Bynum, the twentieth century has been dominated by laboratory medicine – that the understanding of the mechanisms of a disease is established by the practices within a laboratory, and the diagnosis of a patient's disease is similarly achieved by extracting substances of the patient (through blood samples, urine, biopsies etc.) that can be investigated within the same laboratory regime. Even therapies are created at the laboratory, for example by developing drugs such as factor VIII (Bynum 2008; see also Keating and Cambrioso 2006). For researchers such as Curran and Jaffe, the laboratory also includes methods and theories that are combined in a way to move knowledge forward. According to science historian Hans-Jörg Rheinberger (1997), the practices within a laboratory are based on different types of experimental systems that researchers create and maintain within their specific laboratory. Experimental system refers to a system within a laboratory consisting of both methods and theories that allows the researcher to find new answers in regard to the phenomena that the researcher wants to investigate. These systems consist of advanced laboratory instruments that monitor the phenomena, different forms of hosts or organs and other tools, competences and infrastructure that are necessary to conduct their research. Both Harold Jaffe and James Curran point out that they were arguing about which experimental systems (or model) they should use at the CDC, a system developed to study gonorrhea or a system focusing on hepatitis. As the quote above suggests, hemophilia patients made it apparent for the researchers to choose an experimental system that resembled the hepatitis system, instead of gonorrhea.

Similarly, Mangalasseril G. Sarngadharan, who was working at a biomedical laboratory, regarded the cases of hemophilia patients as a clue that narrowed the search for what the infection was that caused AIDS. They speculated that it had to be some sort of retrovirus, like HTLV:

> It had to be a virus, there were things like people getting infected by taking factor VIII, which is a filtered product ... if it's filtered it shouldn't have any bacteria or cells in there.
>
> (FoA: 2003_9_02)

Knowing how factor VIII was manufactured (with filters), the researchers at laboratories were guided in their search through the events and the cases taking place in hospitals – and the occurrence of AIDS among people with hemophilia narrowed the search for an explanation.

In 1981–1982, laboratory medicine, as described by Bynum, was still trying to catch up with the discoveries that the doctors made in the hospital regarding AIDS. Including hemophilia into the picture was a clue, pushing researchers and physicians in the right direction. The hemophilia patients were with their bodies and their dependency of factor VIII like advanced laboratory instruments outside of the laboratory that filtered some of the noise in the process of trying to understand the disease, through their tragedy of falling victims of the virus.

"They were the victims, they were the ones, we felt sorry for"

However, the narrative of hemophilia within the story of AIDS also provides, based on the interviews in the FoA, a political/societal dimension. People with hemophilia were affected by the ways society reacted to AIDS, especially in the United States. The strong association between AIDS and gay sex created mistrust and skepticism from the hemophilia community when the findings were initially presented.

As Philip Pizzo stated, "In the beginning there was a lot of denial that this was in any way related to the syndrome that had been described in homosexual gay men" (FoA: 2006_7_04). For the researchers at CDC, James Curran and Harold Jaffe, this became even more strenuous. Harold Jaffe recalled a meeting in Atlanta in January 1983 that they organized to present to:

> the blood banking community and the doctors who treat hemophilia the evidence that we had. That whatever it was, was in the blood supply and our feeling was we proved it and the discussions should be what should we do about it.... We were astonished and very disappointed to discover that the blood bankers simply didn't accept this. I remember one of them saying well you convinced us that there is some odd disease going on here but I don't think it is the same disease, and their attitude was that until you convince us we're not going to do anything and they didn't do anything.
>
> (FoA: 2007_40)

Despite the reluctant initial response, the realization that blood, and especially the blood supplies, could be infected and transmit the disease created attention. While the hemophilia foundations were hesitant, many governments internationally pushed for guidelines that in retrospect limited the historic epidemic, even though they at times included a temporary ban on gay men donating blood (many studies have focused on the international variation of blood bank governance and limitations; see Feldman 1999; Steffen 1999; Gilmore and Somerville 1999; Albæk 1999; 2001; Dressler 1999; Izzo 1999; Ballard 1999; Berner 2007; 2012). The hemophilia community, with their reliance on large quantities of blood, as described by Larry Kramer, created a strong bond of trust and dependency between the patient groups and the blood banks and pharmaceutical companies. Thus, this community was reluctant to stop blood banks or to create a moratorium with the risk of losing their only really effective drug.

The cases of people with hemophilia as well as cases of patients infected through blood transfusion also attracted attention to the epidemic that was on the brink of exploding. Harold Jaffe argued that:

> Media wasn't interested and wrote very little about it, it wasn't until the end of 1982 that they suddenly became very interested because that's when we started learning about cases with transfusion and cases in young infants.
>
> (FoA: 2007_40)

James Curran similarly experienced that the budget started to increase when there were concerns that AIDS was in the blood supplies, when the epidemic could be a more generalized one.

> It became apparent for America that the cause of AIDS could affect virtually anyone through a blood transfusion for example that there was a wide spread risk and the wide spread risk that said to America that this could happen to me.
>
> (FoA: 2006_10)

With the cases of AIDS among people with hemophilia, society started to pay attention to what was going on. As Alvin Friedman-Kien comments:

> It wasn't until the hemophiliacs became infected and they acquired AIDS ... *they were the victims, they were the ones, we felt sorry for* and it was then the government, the CDC and everybody else got very very concerned, especially the NIH, about this epidemic that was affecting people through blood and blood products.
>
> (FoA: 2007_41, emphasis by author)

Hence, with cases of people with hemophilia, government, media and the entire population of America started to take the disease seriously. Once it started to affect blood supplies, it also affected everyone.

"Afraid of the plague"

Once the attention of the population finally was created, it quickly spun out of control – the hemophilia narrative also reveals the crude and evil behavior of people. Any behavior that deviates from any perception of a clear norm (whatever that norm might be) can lead to stigmatization. Whereas gay men suffered from stigmatization based on their sexuality, people with hemophilia had suffered from stigmatization owing to their "fragility" and often deformations caused by their hereditary disease. With the fear of AIDS people with hemophilia experienced a stigma upon a stigma. James Curran noted:

> It's remarkable that persons from hemophilia that had AIDS & HIV infection were also discriminated against. It was not just homosexuality and drug use that were causing the discrimination it was the disease itself. People were afraid of AIDS and they were afraid of contamination they didn't want Ryan White to go to their school – they burnt down the house of three hemophiliac boys in Florida because they were *afraid of the plague.*
>
> (FoA: 2006_10, emphasis by author)

Shortly after it became known to the society at large, being identified with HIV/AIDS was by many an acceptable cause for exclusion. Children were banned from kindergartens and playgrounds; they were shunned and avoided at every cost. In the citation of James Curran, he refers to two names, Ryan White and the Ray brothers (FoA: 2007_america_and_aids_edited; FoA: 2006_7_04). These children not only became victims of the disease but also victims of their communities. Families and officials banned Ryan White from school where they lived after being informed that he had HIV. Ryan White and his mother had to move to another state in order for him to go to school.

Ricky Ray and his two brothers were similarly banned from school and shunned by their community in Arcadia, Florida. News coverage, aired in July 1987 and available today on YouTube, gives an immediate, emotional impression of their case. The voice-over describes the three boys as normal lively young-sters (at that time eight, nine and eleven years old), treated like lepers of old. The Baptist pastor (Raul Gamiotea) in their village even banned the family from church and warned other community members of the family's disease. The family decided to sue the school and, after the court overruled the decision to ban the three boys, they were admitted to school only to become victims of arson, since someone decided to burn down their home. In the news coverage Clifford Ray, emotionally affected by the treatment of his sons, commented:

> They are going to have to look back one day and I don't think it is far in the future, they will look back and say: we treated them young men wrong and there will be nothing they can do but to hang their head in shame.
>
> (https://youtu.be/SRfIb5TpMmg)

These cases became famous as tragic yet crucial milestones in the hemophilia/ AIDS narrative, not in their misfortune but in the actions, activism and "sober-ing" of civil society that these cases forced the U.S. government and society to do. Ryan White became good friends with celebrities such as Elton John and Michael Jackson, and eventually Bill Clinton signed the Ryan White CARE act to assist people with HIV/AIDS. Similarly, Congress passed a Relief Act in 1998, named after Ricky Ray, to subsidize health care for people with hemo-philia that were suffering from HIV/AIDS. These governmental actions were the result of pressure from activists. As Alvin Friedman-Kien concludes:

> The people who were most active most helpful were the people who were relatives and foundations that were dedicated to hemophilia and to blood and blood products once the blood banks in this country realized that they were infected this became a very major issue.
>
> (FoA: 2007_41)

It is beyond the scope of this chapter to analyze the effects that the gay com-munity and the hemophilia community had on each other. But looking at these communities, and how they are documented in the Face of AIDS film archive one starts to speculate that these two groups learned a lot from each other and that the strength of the AIDS community is a result of the juxtaposition of both gay activists and the hemophilia patient organizations. In an interview posted on YouTube by the HIV story project in San Francisco, Clifford Ray says:

> If it wasn't for the gay community my family would be in a worse condition than they were. It was the gay community that stepped up and got behind us when we were down and out. When we had nowhere else to live it was the gay community that found us somewhere to live. Our religious beliefs and the friends we made in the gay community had to go hand in hand. We still love them and care about everyone of them – they stepped forward and helped us.
>
> (https://youtu.be/vrZwdTvaXVM)

Paradoxically, it might have been the combination of, on the one hand, a community of activists, distrusting the society at large and the authorities, with their willingness to fight against officials to get their rights, and, on the other, a community working on the inner lines of the pharmaceutical and health care systems that determined the relatively rapid response to AIDS.

Conclusion: from interview to film to paper

Even though people with hemophilia were victims of HIV/AIDS they did not remain victims, at least not according to the stories available in the Face of AIDS film archive. They were primarily instrumental in a couple of milestones, such as narrowing the possible patterns of how this sexually transmitted disease behaved, forcing the population to be concerned about the disease and ultimately caring about those living with the virus.

This narrative, available in the Face of AIDS film archive, was also presented in the film that was produced by Staffan Hildebrand. The film especially focused on the mobilizing forces that Ryan White and others created, which in turn lead to systemized forms of health care within the U.S. system. By combining some of the voices available in the archive with images of Ryan White (for example), a very compelling narrative is created in the film where these individuals bring a positive conclusion to an otherwise tragic story. Since many of the interviews marked with hemophilia A were used in this film it might not be surprising that the film confirms the account that I could make from the same interviews. However, the interviews and the backdrop of medical history and other history related to HIV and hemophilia, as well as the accounts on YouTube, enable me to describe the differences between the Face of AIDS film archive and other traditional archives. Where both forms of archives have different strength and weaknesses, the first allows emotions and wide assumptions; the other enables us to dwell on details and differences.

I would like to conclude by returning to Larry Kramer's speculations in the beginning of this chapter. It is probably is farfetched to argue that gay people with hemophilia spread the disease after obtaining it through factor VIII. However, people with hemophilia suffered immensely during the first decade of AIDS. In Sweden, more than 100 persons with hemophilia contracted HIV through American factor VIII drugs. This was one fifth of the entire Swedish hemophilia population at that time. The way blood was collected; the way plasma was pooled together before factor VIII was extracted increased the risk of infection significantly. In this sense, Larry Kramer is right that the pharmaceutical companies neglected the risk and exposed an entire community to the virus.

In contrast to the dystopian remarks by Larry Kramer, maybe it is also fair to argue that people with hemophilia who contracted the HIV virus from their treatment resulted in a shift both for the research efforts of trying to understand the disease as well as a sobering of fear and stigmatization within society at large, especially manifested in the two bills that were signed by Congress. However, perhaps the strongest (positive?) consequence of the way AIDS affected both the gay and hemophilia community was how they merged as what David Kirp described as an "odd couple" (Kirp 1999). The impact these two communities had on each other and on society, the government and the pharmaceutical industry probably resides in the delicate balance between trust and distrust, dependency and activism, that has become significant for the rise of informed patients movements (Epstein 1996).

Note

1 I have written about the development of factor VIII in Sweden elsewhere (Normark, 2015). In Sweden, the factor was first purified by Birger and Margareta Blombäck in 1954 (Blombäck and Blombäck 1956; Blombäck, B. 2007; Blombäck, M. 2007; 2011a), which in turn led to treatment for hemophilia A (Nilsson, Blombäck, Blombäck and Ramgren 1962). At first the fractioning process of blood was conducted in the basement of the chemistry department at Karolinska Institutet but moved to a pilot plant within the campus in 1960 before Kabi AB (a pharmaceutical company) was finally convinced to produce the antihemophilic factor on industrial scale in 1967 (for a detailed description of the process see Jorpes, Blombäck, Blombäck and Magnusson 1962).

References

Albæk, Erik (1999). "The Never-Ending Story? The Political and Legal Controversies over HIV and the Blood Supply in Denmark," in Eric Feldman and Ronald Bayer (eds.), *Blood Feuds: AIDS, Blood and the Politics of Medical Disaster*, pp. 161–190. Oxford: Oxford University Press.

Albæk, Erik (2001). "Managing Crisis: HIV and the Blood Supply" and "Protecting the Swedish Blood Supply against HIV: Crisis Management without Scandal," in Mark Bovens, Paul Hart and Guy Peters (eds.), *Success and Failure in Public Governance*, pp. 453–469 and pp. 551–566. Northampton: Edward Elgar.

Ballard, John (1999). "HIV-Contaminated Blood and Australian Policy: The Limits of Success," in Eric Feldman and Ronald Bayer (eds.), *Blood Feuds: AIDS, Blood and the Politics of Medical Disaster*, pp. 243–270. Oxford: Oxford University Press.

Bayer, Ronald (1999). "Blood and AIDS in America: Science, Politics and the Making of an Iatrogenic Catastrophe," in Eric Feldman and Ronald Bayer (eds.), *Blood Feuds: AIDS, Blood and the Politics of Medical Disaster*, pp. 19–58. Oxford: Oxford University Press.

Berner, Boel (2012). *Blodflöden: Blodgivning och blodtransfusion i det svenska samhället*. Lund: Arkiv förlag.

Berner, Boel (2007). "Understanding the Contaminated Blood Affair. The Uses of Cross-National Comparisons," *Health, Risk and Society*, 9(1): 105–112.

Blombäck, Birger (2007). "A Journey with Bleeding Time Factor" in Giorgio Semenza (ed.), *Stories of Success: Personal Recollections, X*, pp. 209–255. Amsterdam and Oxford: Elsevier.

Blombäck, Birger and Margareta Blombäck (1956). "Purification of Human and Bovine Fibrogen," *Arkiv för kemi*, 10(29): 415–443.

Blombäck, Margareta (2007). "Thrombosis and Hemostasis Research: Stimulating, Hard Work and Fun," *Thrombosis and Hemostasis*, 98: 8–15.

Blombäck, Margareta (2011a). *Blood Coagulation Research at Karolinska Institutet 1920–2004 PART I – Basic Research*. Published on May 8, 2011, Karolinska Institutet 200 years anniversary.

Blombäck, Margareta (2011b). *Blood Coagulation Research at Karolinska Institutet 1956–2004 PART II – Clinical Research*. Published on May 8, 2011, Karolinska Institutet 200 years anniversary.

Bovens, Mark, Paul Hart and Guy Peters (2001). *Success and Failure in Public Governance*. Northampton: Edward Elgar.

Bynum, William F. (2008). *The History of Medicine: A Very Short Introduction*. Oxford: Oxford University Press.

Dressler, Stephan (1999). "Blood 'Scandal' and AIDS in Germany," in Eric Feldman and Ronald Bayer (eds.), *Blood Feuds: AIDS, Blood and the Politics of Medical Disaster*, pp. 191–212. Oxford: Oxford University Press.

Epstein, S. (1996). *Impure Science: AIDS, Activism, and the Politics of Knowledge*. Berkeley, CA: University of California Press.

Feldman, Eric (1999). "HIV and Blood in Japan: Transforming Private Conflict into Public Scandal," in Eric Feldman and Ronald Bayer (eds.), *Blood Feuds: AIDS, Blood and the Politics of Medical Disaster*, pp. 59–94. Oxford: Oxford University Press.

Feldman, Eric and Ronald Bayer (1999). *Blood Feuds: AIDS, Blood and the Politics of Medical Disaster*. Oxford: Oxford University Press.

Garrett, Laurie (1994). *The Coming Plague: Newly Emerging Diseases in a World Out of Balance*. New York: Farrar, Straus and Giroux.

Gilmore, Norbert and Margaret Somerville (1999). "From Trust to Tragedy: HIV/AIDS and the Canadian Blood System," in Eric Feldman and Ronald Bayer (eds.), *Blood Feuds: AIDS, Blood and the Politics of Medical Disaster*, pp. 127–160. Oxford: Oxford University Press.

Izzo, Umberto (1999). "Blood Bureaucracy and Law: Responding to HIV-Tainted Blood in Italy," in Eric Feldman and Ronald Bayer (eds.), *Blood Feuds: AIDS, Blood and the Politics of Medical Disaster*, pp. 213–242. Oxford: Oxford University Press.

Jorpes, Erik, Birger Blombäck, Margareta Blombäck and Staffan Magnusson (1962). "A Pilot Plant for the Preparation of a Human Plasma Fraction Containing the Human Antihaemophilic Factor A (Factor VIII) and v. Willebrand's Factor," *Acta Medica Scandinavia*, 171(Supplementum 379): 7–21.

Karolinska Sjukhuset (1996). *Blödarsjuka, från Arosenius till nu och framtid*. Karolinska Sjukhuset lär ut, 21/4 1996.

Keating, Peter and Alberto Cambrosio (2006). *Biomedical Platforms: Realigning the Normal and the Pathological in Late Twentieth-Century Medicine*. Cambridge, MA: MIT.

Kirp, David (1999). "The Politics of Blood: Hemophilia Activism in the AIDS Crisis," in Eric Feldman and Ronald Bayer (eds.), *Blood Feuds: AIDS, Blood and the Politics of Medical Disaster*, pp. 293–322. Oxford: Oxford University Press.

McLuhan, Marshall (2003). *Understanding Media: The Extensions of Man*. Critical ed. Corte Madera, CA: Gingko Press.

Nilsson, Inga Maria, Margareta Blombäck, Birger Blombäck and Olof Ramgren (1962). "The Use of Human AHF (Fraction I-O) in Haemophilia A," *Blut*, 8: 92–101.

Nilsson, Inga Marie, Birger Blombäck, Margareta Blombäck and Sven Svennerud (1956). "Kvinnlig hämofili och dess behandling med humant antihämofiliglobulin," *Nordisk Medicin*, 56: 1654–1662.

Normark, Daniel (2015). "Clotting Processes: Stabilization and Destabilization of Roles and Organizations in the Development of a Treatment of Haemophilia," paper presented as part of the session on Ownership and Professionalism: Examples from Swedish Education and Higher Education, 1945–2010 at the 4S/ESOCITE Conference, August 20–23, in Buenos Aires, Argentina.

Rheinberger, Hans-Jörg (1997). *Toward a History of Epistemic Things: Synthesizing Proteins in the Test Tube.* Stanford, CA: Stanford University Press.

Sköld, Erik (1944). *On Hæmophilia in Sweden and Its Treatment by Blood Transfusion.* Stockholm: P.A. Norstedt & söner.

Steffen, Monika (1999). "The Nation's Blood: Medicine, Justice, and the State in France," in Eric Feldman and Ronald Bayer (eds.), *Blood Feuds: AIDS, Blood and the Politics of Medical Disaster*, pp. 95–126. Oxford: Oxford University Press.

Stormorken, Helge (2005). *Paul A. Owren: The Golden Era of Haemostasis.* Oslo: Gazettebok.

Part II

Aesthetics, representations, narratives

5 Performativity and documentary aesthetics in Staffan Hildebrand's earliest conference films on AIDS in the 1980s

Tommy Gustafsson

The performative documentary

Documentaries have, since their institutional inception during the 1930s, been perceived as more educational and truthful than fictional feature films and television productions. Correspondingly, documentary film theory has been preoccupied with the question of truth, that is, how different types of documentaries function aesthetically and stylistically in relation to "reality" and the real-life world that they purport to explain and portray (see, for example, Nichols 2010; Winston 2013). This durable focus on reality has in an unfortunate way created an epistemological understanding of the documentary genre where the historical development of the genre seems to strive for an ever more realistic way to transfer reality and truth to film.

An important reason for this is the fact that the study of the documentary film is underdeveloped on a theoretical level. Bill Nichols's five documentary modes – poetic, expository, participatory, observational, reflexive – have had a more or less solitary influence on the contemporary study of the documentary film genre. In recent years, this dominant way of understanding the documentary genre has been challenged, among others by film scholar Stella Bruzzi, who has criticized these modes for not providing an understanding of documentary films on a more complex level. Instead, these modes just become boxes where very different films are placed or squeaked in without sufficient clarifications (Bruzzi 2006: 1–8).

Bruzzi's foremost contribution to documentary film theory is an elaboration of performativity, in alignment with philosopher Judith Butler's theory of gender performativity, but connecting the performative element to artistic means and choices instead of gender. According to Bruzzi, a documentary film becomes performative when it makes sense of the interaction between performance and reality. That is, a performative documentary is a continuous act of negotiation between the filmmaker and "reality." Performativity, in the Bruzzian sense, can therefore be seen as a way to undermine the conventional documentary's pursuit of truth and representations of reality. Performativity can also be seen as an approach where you simply look for the subjective by considering the objective as a utopia that cannot be achieved. The emphasizing of performative elements thus becomes a way of recognizing the documentary genre's instability (Bruzzi 2006: 8, 153–180).

In response to this criticism, Nichols created a sixth mode, called the performative mode, which is another documentary narrative that appears in the 1980s, chronologically after the other five modes. Nichols, in stark contrast to Bruzzi, believes that performative documentaries primarily address us emotionally and with emotional arguments rather than with facts and evidence, and, consequently, as less-true documentaries. The intention is to place the audience in a subjective position, in line with the film's specific perspective on the world, i.e., female perspective, gay perspective, class perspective. According to Nichols, the performative documentary tries to represent a social subjectivity that connects the specific with the general, the individual with the collective, and the personal with the political (Nichols 2010: 200–211).

Although performativity is a way to undermine the conventional documentary's pursuit of truth, using emotional arguments, rather than evidence, could create an even more powerful type of documentary. This is due to the fact that the smallest common denominator for documentaries is not truth, or honesty, as Bruzzi denotes it (155), but instead the circumstance that a documentary, regardless of its subject, mode, or subgenre, needs to have a relation to the real world. That is, the aspect of reality that the documentary filmmaker wants to portray or analyze has to either have happened (historical documentaries) or be about a social subject or a real-life person (contemporary documentaries), otherwise it is a mockumentary or a fictional film. These two performative perspectives open up new ways of analyzing and understanding documentaries.

One of those aspects is the fact that the documentary genre is not clinically separated from other film genres in, for instance, the use of music, animated sequences, or editing. Bruzzi and Nichols both point to numerous examples of documentaries that, stylistically, dissolve genre boundaries. However, while Bruzzi interprets this as liberating for the documentary genre, Nichols perceives it as a loss of credibility. This, in turn, opens up the tricky proximity between the documentary film and the fiction film.

Here I would like to develop the idea of this proximity and the synergies that exist between the documentary genre and the fictional film/television concerning how audiences understood such a subject as AIDS in the 1980s. Staffan Hildebrand's early conference films, *AIDS: föreställningar om en verklighet* ("AIDS: Perceptions about a Reality," 1986) and *Crossover: The Global Impact of AIDS* (1988), are both, of course, documentaries, but they are also information films. Furthermore, *Crossover* was made in two versions, both as a twenty-minute conference film and a fifty-two-minute television version that was broadcast by Discovery Channel U.S.A., SVT (Swedish public television), and Australian television, among others (Hildebrand 2017: 1). What is more, these films were not made in a cultural vacuum. First, Hildebrand had made several films before, both documentaries and genre films, mostly focusing on topics that concerned Swedish youth and adolescence, including the highly successful youth film *G – som i gemenskap* ("C – as in Community," 1983). It is not an unreasonable thought that aesthetics from his previous films and documentaries found their way into these documentary films. Hence, I will add an auteur perspective, seldom used in documentary film theory, to enhance and understand the performative elements in Hildebrand's filmmaking. Second, according to Paula A. Treichler, AIDS is a story primarily read from the body of the homosexual man (1999: 37), and the homosexual man was still an anomaly in mainstream film and television in the early 1980s.

I will pose three interrelated research questions in this chapter: (1) How does Hildebrand frame, portray, and explain the notion of AIDS aesthetically and stylistically in relation to his previous films and a Swedish tradition of information films? (2) How do Hildebrand's conference films relate to global and mainstream images of the homosexual man in the early 1980s? (3) From a performative perspective, in what ways, if any, does the documentary genre in general synergize with fictional film and television?

Media images of AIDS in the early 1980s

How does the public understand and make sense of a new epidemic such as AIDS? Roughly, two main discourses can be distinguished in the early 1980s, a medical and a medial. These two discourses are not separated. Medical information can and is transferred via different mass media such as documentary films or television programs. The media can, and does, use medical information in their stories but mass media, obviously, does not have any obligations to be accurate and true to that information but can modify it for aesthetic or commercial reasons. Furthermore, media outlets have different intentions for the spread of information, knowledge, and opinions (Hadenius and Weibull 2005: 165, 176). Swedish public television has, for example, an obligation to keep a neutral and informed tone, while big U.S. television networks have commercial obligations, and private religious media outlets such as *Old Time Gospel Hour* (1956–), founded by televangelist Jerry Falwell, maintains a "Christian" agenda that affects the broadcast information.

Still, audiovisual productions about AIDS tend to obtain an educational value just because of their grave subject, regardless of its interpretation. Many films with an AIDS theme deal with the history of the epidemic in question, usually with the intention to teach their audiences, which is often the case with documentaries, but this didactic tone also occurs in feature films, for example in *Philadelphia* (Jonathan Demme, 1993). Both documentaries and feature films thus affect the knowledge of their audiences, perhaps by enhancing an already existing memory taught in school or elsewhere or by introducing fresh knowledge where audiences learn something new, which potentially was the case with regard to AIDS in the early 1980s. This new knowledge can then be dismissed, altered, or confirmed, e.g., via repetition in other documentary films and television programs on AIDS or by other sources of information, such as schools, churches, or news reporting.

The knowledge about AIDS in the early 1980s was characterized by uncertainty, both as a medical concern but also in the news media and, thus, by the public. As science reporter Lawrence M. Altman recalled, "at the time, we had little idea what we were dealing with – didn't know that AIDS was a distinct disease, what caused it, how it could be contracted, or even what to call it" (Altman 2011). However, early on AIDS was connected to "the gay lifestyle" and the disease was for a short period know as GRID, "gay-related immune deficiency." In an early newscast on *NBC Nightly News* AIDS was reported as a form of "cancer" and it was said that "the scientists say that this probably means they are dealing with a new *deadly* sexual transmitted disease" (emphasis by the news anchor). The news segment mentioned that a few heterosexuals had been infected but interviewed only homosexual men with AIDS (NBC 1982), thus clearly placing the focus on gay men. What was called the AIDS scare or AIDS hysteria grew out of this uncertainty, and a lack of public education. There are numerous examples of how this created reactions, and discrimination, such as keeping children home from school, firing people with HIV/AIDS from their jobs, or refusing to give medical assistance owing to the fear of catching the disease.

Critics have compared the AIDS scare to the era of anti-Communist paranoia in the U.S. in the 1950s (see for example Phair 1986). Despite almost daily reporting about AIDS in newspapers and on television around the western hemisphere in the mid-1980s, there were still a lot of people who were misinformed about the disease and how it was transmitted. The fact that it was incurable, and connected to moral imperatives about the "gay lifestyle," was something that scientists had to combat. However, this was also an excuse for religious authorities to impose alternative truths and "cures," such as abstinence; since homosexuality was seen as sin and AIDS as the punishment (see, for example, YLE 1993). Even so, Treichler points out that the first decade of mainstream media representations of AIDS were "safe, clichéd, heterosexist pieties that largely reproduced conventional humanist orthodoxies" and that this in fact contributed to hinder "overt extremist hysteric [and] homophobic quarantine" (1999: 124).

In light of these, then, still awakening, and somewhat alarmist discussions of AIDS, who were the first faces of AIDS in Hildebrand's films and how did he choose to portray an epidemic that had relatively few previous points of cinematic references?

Performativity and the aesthetics of AIDS in Hildebrand's films

Staffan Hildebrand's first two conference films, *AIDS: föreställningar om en verklighet* and *Crossover: The Global Impact of AIDS*, are, at a first glance, very different. *AIDS: föreställningar om en verklighet* is a short, seventeen-minute low-budget documentary shot in Stockholm, Sweden, while *Crossover* has a much larger budget and is shot on five continents and in nine different countries. Moreover, *Crossover* has well-known American actor Martin Sheen as the all-knowing narrator, adding both credibility, gravity, and international flair to the depictions of AIDS, while *AIDS: föreställningar om en verklighet* is shot in Swedish with Hildebrand himself as the narrator. Yet both documentaries have great similarities in their aesthetic choices and the themes that the films promote, which

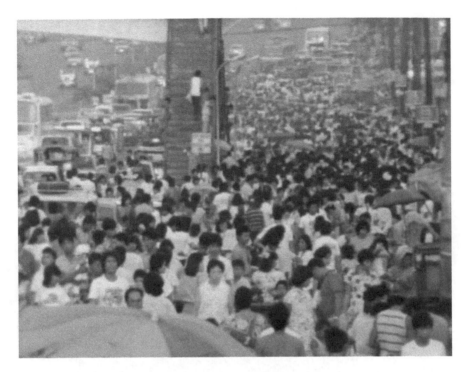

Figure 5.1 Anonymous people around the world. *Crossover*.
Source: Hildebrand, 1988.

point to performative qualities that reach beyond relying on facts and the mere truth. Both films do have the mutual message that the AIDS epidemic is "a worldwide issue which concerns everyone regardless of their sexual preferences" (FoAFA: a).

AIDS: föreställningar om en verklighet and *Crossover* both begin with collages of moving images underlined by cautious ominous scores. In the first case, we see anonymous people in the Stockholm subway filmed in slow motion followed by a magnified image of the virus and then the title. In the latter case, we have two versions. In the longer television version of *Crossover*, aimed at general audiences, the collage consists of locations and anonymous people from the U.S.A., Asia, Africa, Europe, South America, and Australia, followed by the title, while Martin Sheen delivers, rhythmically, the following preface:

> Something has happened. There is a new deadly disease, which is now spreading all over the world. What is it? How does it affect us? How is it spread? What can the scientist do? What can nations do? Can we protect the young generation? Can mankind change its sexual behavior? Can we stop the drugs? Can we match the challenge? Only the future will tell.
>
> (*Crossover*, 1988)

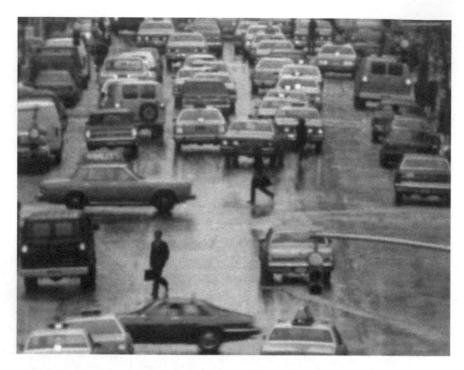

Figure 5.2 Anonymous people around the world. *Crossover*.
Source: Hildebrand, 1988.

In the short conference version of *Crossover* we get, somewhat paradoxically, a "television version," that is, an introduction which uses faster editing of ten talking heads delivering short soundbites ("Sex, drugs and rock n' roll, that party is over"/"It is not a homosexual disease"/"The only way to get AIDS is if you're a homo!"/"AIDS is death") of what is to come, without the ominous score, followed by the title. Then Sheen starts to recite the same text as above to a collage of long shots of world locations and close-ups of anonymous people, and sometimes the images of these faces go into freeze-frame, as of the boy in the ending of *The 400 Blows* (*Les Quatre Cents Coups*, François Truffaut, 1959), which is followed by a second appearance of the title.

The use of slow motion and freeze-frames, an ominous score, and the God-like voice-over all contribute to create a sense of a stealthy threat, as if anyone in the masses could be infected or is in fact already infected, knowingly or not – all according to general knowledge of AIDS among the public at the time.

After the intro, the first film, *AIDS: föreställningar om en verklighet*, is structured into six main segments:

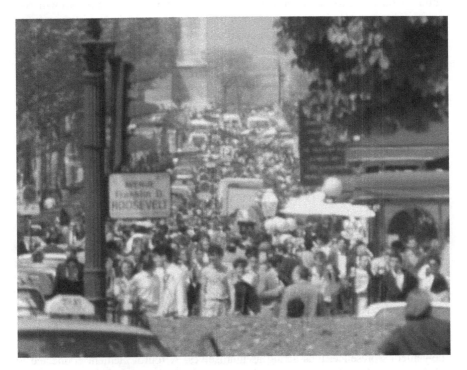

Figure 5.3 Anonymous people around the world. *Crossover.*
Source: Hildebrand, 1988.

1   general information about AIDS from scientists, but where foremost homo-
    sexual men, bisexual people, and drugs users are discussed as bridges to the
    general population;
2   threatening collage where anonymous people in Stockholm are filmed on
    the street in slow motion, of whom several actually look into the camera,
    mixed with superimposed newspaper headlines of the infection;
3   information segment where talking heads criticize the media for sensational-
    ist reporting on the epidemic;
4   interviews with four people who live with HIV: three men and a woman;
5   yet another threat sequence where Hildebrand surreptitiously films
    anonymous people at Café Opera, the most trendy night club in Stockholm
    in the mid-1980s;
6   information segment that concentrates on the question of what safe sex
    constitutes.

Information about AIDS, delivered by experts in an expository way, is thus
interspersed with performative segments that emphasize an invisible threat to the

public. Consequently, this setup runs the risk of holding the first known risk groups – homo- and bisexual people and drug users (of which the only one interviewed is a female sex worker) – accountable for the potential spread of a deadly epidemic. However, the fourth segment, which consists of interviews with Swedish people living with HIV, disrupts this pattern, partly because Hildebrand uses a passive interview technique that lets the subjects themselves, after a while, define their own (sexual) identity, and partly because one of the subjects is a woman who never reveals how she got the virus, leaving it open for interpretation that she could be heterosexual, homosexual, bisexual, hemophiliac, or a previous drug user and/or sex worker.

Going back to Hildebrand's previous documentaries, we can detect a number of aesthetic strategies and how they have developed. In *Fjortonårslandet* ("In the Land of Fourteen-Year-Olds," 1979), a film about different fractions of youth culture in Sweden, the film starts with the same television collage as in the short version of *Crossover*, a sort of declaration of contents. In addition to this we have a narrator, the adolescent Micke, who is part of the youth culture presented in the film, who reads from a screenplay written by Hildebrand, similar to Sheen's reading, thus with the same intention, to give credibility and nowness to what is shown. These recurrent voice-overs are also the voice of the auteur Hildebrand. In addition, credibility is achieved through the passive interview technique later used in *AIDS: föreställningar om en verklighet*, even enhanced by letting the camera roll in order to capture a slice of life, although it is obvious that the subjects are fully aware of the camera's presence, thus acting as themselves. A fourth element connected to this is the use of music to create emotions and to mark modernity, even if the choice of progressive rock band Camel's song "Echoes" (1978) does not, perhaps, equal the teen culture of the late 1970s. The use of music, often scores, in documentary films is common practice, but the use of music also constitutes a break with Nichols's conservative way to place documentaries into different modes according to their ability to stay "clean" when depicting and relating to truth and reality (Nichols 2010: 72–76). Music is therefore a primarily emotional argument, and when used on a personal/auteur level it also becomes a performative element.

These performative elements are further developed in his next film, *Veckan då Roger dödades* ("The Week When Roger Was Killed," 1981), which is a docudrama about a medially noted manslaughter involving young people where Hildebrand uses interviews with relatives, mixed with reenactments based on police and witnesses' reports. The line between reality and performance is obscured by the use of docudrama aesthetics such as literary and narrative techniques to flesh out the bare facts of an event, and the practice to take the license to enhance minor facts for the sake of drama (Paget 2011: 94–130). Furthermore, several of the subjects who are portrayed in *Fjortonårslandet* are used as reenactments actors in *Veckan då Roger dödades*, and this documentary transgression all comes together in the fiction film *G – som i gemenskap*, where the same "unknown" persons now are the actual stars.

In the longer television version of *Crossover*, audiences get a geographically structured account of AIDS, which is in line with the documentary's global intention and reach. After the introduction, where the use of ominous music, slow motion images of anonymous people, and Martin Sheen's voice-over runs the risk of holding risk groups such as homosexual people and drug users accountable, Hildebrand twists this perspective. *Crossover* is structured into the following seven main segments:

1   The Bronx (U.S.A.) is portrayed as a war zone, focusing on drugs and poverty among African Americans, but in a segment a white woman appears, who blames her infection on her own promiscuity.
2   In Europe (France, Italy), focus is on the young, discussing safe sex and condoms, which is controversial in these Catholic parts of the world. The segment ends with an interview with a young, heterosexual and infected (via drug injection) couple, who answers a question about what they want to tell young people in the following way: "It is stupid to have it. You don't feel it, you don't feel sick. You can't have children; you can't have sexual relations with people you might like to have with."
3   In Southeast Asia (Thailand, Philippines), focus is on the sex trade, and the fact that (male heterosexual) Americans are spreading the epidemic. Furthermore, focus is also on the young's sex education, where a Philippine teacher teaches abstinence, and that the spread of AIDS is the result of too much Western liberalism, that is, via rock culture and Hollywood films.
4   In Rio de Janeiro (Brazil), focus is on poverty among the youth, and child prostitution among adolescent boys.
5   In Africa (Uganda), focus is on the fact that AIDS is a heterosexual disease in Africa, and that the cure is to never mix sex partners.
6   Australia is mentioned as a "dangerous crossover point for AIDS," that is, from homosexual to heterosexual people.
7   In San Francisco (U.S.A.), focus is on the homosexual sphere, claiming that informational campaigns have managed to impede the spread of AIDS by changing sexual behavior, thus ending the film on a successful note.

The twist is a change of balance where the focus on youth, poverty, drug use, prostitution (involuntary due to drug use and poverty) shifts the focus from a "gay disease" to a global epidemic that not only concerns heterosexuals but is also spread, in different ways, by heterosexuals. It is only in the last two parts where the emphasis on homosexuality resurfaces, first as a "danger" in Australia but then as a positive example in the gay community in San Francisco.

As stated, the focus on youth and youth culture is a recurrent trademark of Hildebrand. Another, more performative element that is used in *Crossover* is the let-the-camera-roll aesthetic, which recreates a sense of reality and nowness in staged scenes that border on actual performance. One example is the rap performed by some African American kids from Bronx, and another is the dance scene filmed at a gay club in Paris, where the male participants are highly aware of the camera. Another example is when Hildebrand interviews a bragging male sex buyer in Thailand, asking if he is not afraid of AIDS, and getting the blatant answer: "No! If you get AIDS you are a homo!!" (which is kept in both the short and long versions of *Crossover*).

However, another perspective that permeates *Crossover* is a seemingly moral streak that preaches not only condom use but also sexual abstinence as (the only) safeguard from AIDS. You could argue that it is the subjects – MDs, scientists, teachers, and other persons in position of power – who deliver this message, but it is Hildebrand's choice to use these moral statements, inserting them into the histories of AIDS that he in fact is creating. These sorts of moralizing pointers, although not specifically about sexual abstention, can also be found in *Fjortonårslandet* and *Veckan då Roger dödades*, where, for example, "video violence" is constructed as an active force in the latter documentary, all according to a moral panic about the then new VCR technology that swept through Sweden in the beginning of the 1980s (Gustafsson and Arnberg 2013, *passim*).

According to sociologist Dorothy Nelkin, documentaries on AIDS in the 1980s tended to personify science, making the scientist a star by a script that featured four ingredients: (1) magnified viral images, (2) music underlining the significance, (3) portraying the AIDS crisis as a puzzle being solved by a detective team, and (4) laboratory footage edited to simulate key moments in the chronology of AIDS (Nelkin through Treichler 1999: 190–191). Besides the use of one image of a magnified viral image in *AIDS: föreställningar om en verklighet*, these are features that Hildebrand does not conform to. In fact, scientists, although providing information, are more framed as social actors than as detective scientists with all the answers.

Sweden has a long tradition of using the media of film and television for information purposes, creating a number of films, documentaries, and infomercials about everything from how to pay your taxes to why dads should take parental leave. A very common ingredient in these types of films has been the use of comedy to persuade the public of their own well-being. Even in the case of a deadly serious problem such as AIDS, comedy was employed. In 1985, the Swedish government set up the authority Aidsdelegationen (the National Commission on AIDS) in order to combat the spread of HIV. The chairman was Gertrud Sigurdsen, minister of health and social affairs, and the National Commission on AIDS conducted an intensive information campaign in which, among other things, they propagated the use of condoms but not the instigation of abstinence, with the use of comedy (Thorsén 2013: 97–101, 385–394). For instance, in the informercial *Aidshockey: kärlek börjar med att man lär känna varandra* ("AIDS Ice Hockey: Love Begins with Friendship," 1988), a woman approaches two men in a bar, picking up one of them and then taking him home. A distributer of morning newspapers sees them go into an apartment, and then overhears what sounds like sex. But, in fact, the couple have dressed in hockey gear and are playing hockey in the living room, all while the text "Love Begins with Friendship. The National Commission on AIDS" is superimposed. This is a clear intertextual reference to the popular television film *Ska vi gå hem till dej eller till mej eller var och en till sitt?* ("Should We Go to Your Place, My Place, or All Alone?" 1973), directed by Lasse Hallström, where two characters play board games, including table ice hockey, when the man cannot get erection. This sense of comedy is not present in Hildebrand's films where instead, as the dark threatening introductions to *AIDS: föreställningar om en verklighet* and *Cross-over* demonstrate, a dire gravity hovers over the representations of AIDS. The main reason for this is probably that these documentaries were aimed at a global audience, mainly consisting of international scientists.

However, looking beyond Hildebrand's corpus of previous documentaries, and the Swedish tradition of information films with a comical flavor, how did Hildebrand choose to portray the main face of AIDS at the time, that is, the homosexual man, in comparison to existing mainstream images of the homo-sexual men in the early 1980s?

Media representations of "the homosexual man" of the 1980s

Homosexuality, and the homosexual man in particular, have been part of Western film culture since the silent age. British film scholar Richard Dyer has, in a historical account of lesbian and homosexual films, claimed that the Swedish film *Vingarna* (*The Wings*, 1916) was probably the first film in the world to include a homosexual theme (Dyer 2003: 8). However, *The Wings* does not belong to the category of films that shows homosexuality openly. Instead, the film presents a subtle image with secret codes, dual motifs, and allusions that only the initiated could decode.

The first film explicitly about homosexual people and homosexuality that was presented to a wider audience is the German instructional film *Anders als die Andern* (*Different from the Others*, 1919). This film was the result of a collabora-tion between sexologist Magnus Hirschfeld and film director Richard Oswald, who specialized in "sensational" instructional films (Kracauer 2004: 44; Gustafsson 2014: 139–140). Produced before the establishment of any documentary codes, the film is a mix of pedagogical, documentary-like segments and a fictional docudrama story about love between two men and its consequences under the threat of criminalization, i.e., blackmail and suicide. The idea that homosexual people were doomed to a life of torment and loneliness would become a recurrent stereotype in popular film, especially after World War II, but this image was actually based on medical literature of the time, in which such outcomes were regarded as "natural" developments of the disease homosexuality (Sullivan 2003: 14–19). Addiction to drugs and/or alcohol thus came to serve as a significant symbol of the homosexu-al's need to alleviate this "natural" loneliness.

In a study about representations of AIDS in American film, Kylo-Patrick R. Hart brings up what he calls the cinematic tradition of Otherness, that is, the incorporation of binary oppositions in the narrative in order to structure (the fic-tional) world. AIDS thus has the tendency to be defined according to the binary opposition of general population/risk groups and consequently as innocent victims/guilty victims (Hart 2000: 15–16).

Gay activism in the 1970s had made it possible for homosexual people to be more open about their sexuality. The start of the AIDS epidemic in the early

1980s thus coincided, somewhat ironically, with new ways of representing homosexual people in film and television that tried to break off from the old stereotypes. At this breaking point several examples surface of the "gay man," such as the Jodie Dallas character (played by Billy Crystal) in *Soap* (1977–1981). Considering the importance and the impact that American popular culture had around the world, and not least in Sweden, with its mere two television channels in the 1980s, these images became central for the understanding of homosexuality and homosexual men. One of the more prominent examples is the gay character Steven Carrington (Al Corley) in the prime-time television series *Dynasty* (1981–1989). Here I will briefly analyze the introduction of Al Corley's character as well as the portrayal of Michael Pierson (Aidan Quinn) in the first prime-time television film on AIDS, *An Early Frost* (1985), before continuing to the question of how Hildebrand's films relate to these global and mainstream images of the homosexual man in the early 1980s.

Steven Carrington, a blond hunk, and initially the only son of wealthy oil patriarch Blake Carrington (John Forsythe), is introduced getting drunk on a plane home from New York. He is flying first class and he is upset about an impersonal wedding invitation he has received from his father. As he gets off the airplane, he finds out that the company limo is there to pick up an employee, and that he is to take a cab to the family estate. Arriving there, he takes the side of his future stepmother, defending her against a snobbish wedding planner, and literally takes over the preparations, demonstrating that he has a deep knowledge about design, decoration, and classical music. From this, audiences can surmize that he is a sympathetic person, that he has trouble with his tycoon father, and that he has interests that could be interpreted as "unmanly."

Further on in the triple episode that launched *Dynasty* on January 12, 1981, it is revealed that the father is afraid that his only son will not provide him with an heir. However, it is not until a great confrontation between father and son that it is revealed that Steven in fact is gay, when the father blurts out, "How the hell can you respect the opinion of a man who puts his hands on another man!" This coming out scene is not scripted from a gay perspective but from a heteronormative perspective, aimed at audiences acquainted with older stereotypical representations of the homosexual man. The father is trying to understand his son, even admitting that "a little homosexual experimentation is acceptable," but when he realizes that this is not a passing phase he gets angry and frustrated, referring (in a didactic way) to the fact that the American Psychiatric Association declassified homosexuality as a mental illness in 1974. Still, he cannot accept Steven's sexual identity and demands that he should "straighten himself out." The fact that homosexuality is not a mental illness thus becomes "proof" of the ability to choose one's sexual identity according to the father's thinking.

Hence, the representation of Steven is built on older stereotypes of homosexual men as "feminine" and as the miserable gay loner using remedies, but the sheer space in the series allows the character to develop over the course of the series, and thus to change some of these stereotypical features.

An Early Frost has been thoroughly analyzed, as a medical drama to educate the public about AIDS in a time when the epidemic was surrounded by uncertainty, rumors, and disdain (see Treichler 1999: 254–278), and as melodrama, where family relations are broken because of the unavoidable coming out act, rather than because of the death sentence that AIDS was at the time. As Hart writes, "[t]he most common representation of gay men in AIDS movies portrays gay men as embarrassments to their parents, particularly their fathers, with whom they have especially strained (or even nonexistent) relationships after they reveal their homosexuality" (Hart 2000: 51). In *An Early Frost*, Michael's father's first reaction is to hit his son after he has revealed his homosexuality, and that conflict parallels the AIDS theme throughout the film. Nevertheless, Aidan Quinn's character is the neat, sensitive stereotype, well-dressed, handsome, and skillful at playing the piano, as was the Steven Carrington character. One enlightening example is the near total lack of physical intimacy between Michael and his longtime partner, Peter (D.W. Moffett), and when they do touch each other the soundtrack repeatedly plays a "Disney-like" jingle with the purpose to negate any sexual intentions (Treichler 1999: 266). Another example is the comic sidekick Victor (John Glover), who dies of AIDS, joking about it until the very end. Hence, historically negative stereotypes are replaced by, seemingly, positive stereotypes.

The homosexual man and AIDS are thus two problematic subjects that merge and reinforce one another in, and with the help of, mainstream media, in the process creating a perceived cohesion among the public. In order to render the old stereotype (sickly, eccentric, possible child molester) harmless, efforts are made to make the homosexual man innocuous. This tendency can be detected in Hildebrand's previous work, most notably in *G – som i gemenskap*, where the bi/gay character Kristoffer appears as one of several guides-to-life for the young characters in the film, who are still searching for their identities. Kristoffer is portrayed as excessively effeminate, almost on the verge of being ridiculous, but the character is played by Swedish popstar Magnus Uggla, known for his real-life cockiness and attitude, which to a certain point counterbalances the effeminacy, generating some disarming humor.

Although balanced in representing the AIDS epidemic as a global concern for both heterosexual and homosexual people, Hildebrand's conference films nevertheless contain a great majority of homosexual men who are sick, worried, or carry the virus. Here the performative choices of subjects, editing, camera angels, framing, settings, music, and interview questions are of utmost importance in order to portray these men. Consciously, and perhaps unconsciously, these portrayals have to compete with both the positive and negative stereotypes of homosexual men present in society and in the mindset of the public.

In *AIDS: föreställningar om en verklighet* the participating homosexual men living with HIV are few and, perhaps most importantly, in an early stage where the virus has not yet led to AIDS. They are also given the opportunity to define their sexual identities. In the television version of *Crossover*, four homosexual men with developed AIDS appear in the introduction, setting a heavy mark as to whom this disease has affected. Three of them are literally dying, and they are all filmed in their hospital beds with the camera at bed level, sometimes with lenses zooming in on their marked faces as they, prompted by Hildebrand's questions, reject their lifestyles of drugs and casual sex. These scenes are without music or other sound effects, but they are intercut with the above-cited text that Martin Sheen recites, coupled with the threatening music and moody milieu images. The only exception is a 15-second-long and uncommented scene taken at a hospital in Uganda, where we can glimpse anonymous men, women, and children dying of AIDS.

The first of the homosexual men, an Australian, is filmed together with a doctor, who briefly explains the disease, talks about "behavior modifications," and is filmed from a frog perspective, as if the patient is looking up at him. This patient is the only one who returns a bit later, this time sitting up, explaining how close to death he has been several times. The scene ends with Sheen's voice declaring that, "ten hours after this interview he died."

There is then a long hiatus, where altogether five drug users with HIV from different paths of life and parts of the world are interviewed, none of whom has developed any visible signs of AIDS. The contrast is devastating, as it has a tendency to counteract the "neutrality" toward AIDS that these films ostensibly embrace. In the final segment, on San Francisco, the focus shifts back to homosexual men, and there are another four people with HIV figuring in this segment. However, only one man is interviewed, while the rest remain in the background as anonymous patients without visible signs of AIDS. The interviewed person reveals that he just got the virus. He is filmed from below, casually hanging over a railing at a restaurant, as if Hildebrand just walked by and switched on the camera. There is, consequently, no tangible correlation between the mainstream images of homosexual men and the documentary constructions found in Hildebrand's early conference films. Nevertheless, the editing, the structuring of segments, and the use of sound sometimes create an ambivalent threat than mainly is connected to the homosexual man.

Concluding discussion

How do you portray and explain an epidemic such as AIDS to audiences without access to previous points of references? Moreover, how do you untangle a story of AIDS that, at the time, was deeply intertwined with an image of the homosexual man, and all stereotypical traits connected to that image? The analysis in this chapter shows that Hildebrand, in his earliest conference films, chose a number of aesthetic and stylistic strategies, whereof many could be traced back to his previous documentary as well as fiction films. The use of "television collage" as a declaration of contents, the use of a voice-over or a narrator that reads from a screenplay obviously written by Hildebrand, the passive interview technique that creates credibility and nowness, and the choice of letting the camera roll in order to capture a slice of life, are some of these strategies that dissolve the strict border between the documentary genre and other film genres.

With these performative strategies, Hildebrand not only departs from a Swedish tradition of information films; he also manages, in large parts, to untangle the strong correlation between AIDS and homosexual men with the intention to deliver the message that the AIDS epidemic is a global issue that concerns everybody, regardless of sexuality. However, the moral imperative, at the time condemning the so-called gay lifestyle, still lingers over these conference films since Hildebrand constantly frames – through music, editing, and interview questions – the AIDS victims, regardless of sexual identity, as fatalities of life-styles that include drugs and promiscuity. Thus, abstinence and the use of condoms are preached, which, it should be mentioned, were the only "solutions" to the AIDS epidemic that existed at the time. In Sweden, however, the National Commission on AIDS did not promote abstinence as a solution. Moreover, this somewhat dystopian perspective meant that Hildebrand did not portray the sci-entist as a star, as could be seen in other international documentaries on AIDS in the 1980s. Only by the end of the television version of *Crossover* is a short collage of scientists in laboratories, but Sheen's narration, scripted by Hilde-brand, negates the possible heroism: "Scientists and medical industries through-out the world are working on the solution of one of the most difficult health problems ever to face mankind. The cure for AIDS is not merely a scientific challenge; it is a race against time."

Even if Hildebrand used a positive stereotype of a gay man in his popular youth film *G – som i gemenskap*, he did not use either positive or negative stereotypes of homosexual men in his documentary films. Nonetheless, AIDS and homosexuality are two subjects that did reinforce each other during the 1980s, and Hildebrand tried to bend them apart, most prominently by giving space to both men and women to whom the virus had been transmitted through drug injections and/or heterosexual intercourse. This, however, opened up for an ambivalence since none of these people, without exception, shows any signs of AIDS, while the homosexual men, in comparison, often showed visible signs of developed AIDS, even in the last stages, thus boomeranging the AIDS epidemic back as a gay disease.

To conclude, the documentary genre is not clinically separated from other fiction film genres. Rather, the documentary genre synergizes with fictional film and television in numerous ways, thus creating understandings of the world that cannot simply be defined as (a single) truth but as different realities. To talk about performative documentaries or modes is to define certain types of films. It would be more fruitful to adopt a performative perspective on the documentary genre in general, a perspective that not only criticizes transgressions but rather embraces and analyzes these transgressions, emphasizing aesthetic and stylistic elements such as editing, the use of music and sound, narration, framing, and images. One way to approach this is through an auteur analysis of films and film-makers, demonstrated in this chapter with Hildebrand's films. Another way is to employ historical and medial contextualization in order to analyze the (problem-atic yet productive) relation between fiction, faction, and documentary, that is, the continuous negotiation act between the filmmaker and reality.

88   *Tommy Gustafsson*

References

Altman, Lawrence K. (2011). "30 Years In, We Are Still Learning From AIDS," *New York Times*, May 30.
Bruzzi, Stella (2006). *New Documentary: A Critical Introduction*. 2nd ed. London: Routledge.
Dyer, Richard (2003). *Now You See It. Studies in Lesbian and Gay Film*. London and New York: Routledge.
Gustafsson, Tommy and Klara Arnberg (2013). *Moralpanik och lågkultur: genus- och mediahistoriska analyser 1900–2012*. Stockholm: Atlas bokförlag.
Gustafsson, Tommy (2014). *Masculinity in the Golden Age of Swedish Cinema: A Cultural Analysis of the 1920s Films*. Jefferson, NC: McFarland.
Hadenius, Stig and Lennart Weibull (2005). *Massmedier: En bok om press, radio & TV*. Stockholm: Albert Bonniers förlag.
Hart, Kylo-Patrick R. (2000). *The AIDS Movie: Representing a Pandemic in Film and Television*. Birmingham, NY: Haworth.
Hildebrand, Staffan (2017). Unpublished filmography. In the possession of the author.
Kracauer, Siegfried (2004). *From Caligari to Hitler: A Psychological History of the German Film*. Princeton, NJ, and Oxford: Princeton University Press.
NBC (1982). *NBC Nightly News* with Robert Bazell, originally aired on June 17, 1982, available on YouTube, www.youtube.com/watch?v=1LKJ5ZzzL0w, last accessed September 18, 2017.
Nichols, Bill (2010). *Introduction to Documentary*. Bloomington and Indianapolis, IN: Indiana University Press.
Paget, Derek (2011). *No Other Way to Tell It: Docudrama on Film and Television*. Manchester: Manchester University Press.
Phair, John (1986). "The Antidote for Aids Hysteria," *Chicago Tribune*, April 2.
Sullivan, Nikki (2003). *A Critical Introduction to Queer Theory*. New York: New York University Press.
Thorsén, David (2013). *Den svenska aidsepidemin: ankomst, bemötande, innebörd*. Uppsala: Uppsala University.
Treichler, Paula A. (1999). *How to Have Theory in an Epidemic: Cultural Chronicles of AIDS*. Durham, NC, and London: Duke University Press.
Winston, Brian, ed. (2013). *The Documentary Film Book*. London: Palgrave Macmillan/BFI.
YLE, *Talking Heads* (1993). "Är aids straffet för ett promiskuöst leverne?" February 1, https://svenska.yle.fi/artikel/2012/11/14/ar-aids-straffet-ett-promiskuost-leverne, last accessed September 18, 2017.

Films and TV productions

Demme, Jonathan, *Philadelphia* (1993).
Dynasty (ABC, 1981–1989).
Erman, John, *An Early Frost* (1985).
Hallström, Lasse, *Ska vi gå hem till dej eller till mej eller var och en till sitt?* (1973).
Hildebrand, Staffan, *Fjortonårslandet* (1979).
Hildebrand, Staffan, *Veckan då Roger dödades* (1981).
Hildebrand, Staffan, *G – som i gemenskap* (1983).
Hildebrand, Staffan, *AIDS: föreställningar om en verklighet* (1986). Face of AIDS Film Archive, Karolinska Institutet, https://faceofaids.ki.se/archive/1986-aids-forestallningar-om-en-verklighet, last accessed September 19, 2017.

Hildebrand, Staffan, *Crossover: The Global Impact of AIDS* (1988) (short version). Face of AIDS Film Archive, Karolinska Institutet, https://faceofaids.ki.se/archive/1988-crossover-short, last accessed September 19, 2017.

Hildebrand, Staffan, *Crossover: The Global Impact of AIDS* (1988) (full version). Face of AIDS Film Archive, Karolinska Institutet, https://faceofaids.ki.se/archive/1988-crossover-long, last accessed September 19, 2017.

Oswald, Richard, *Anders als die Andern* (1919).

Soap (ABC, 1977–1981).

Stiller, Mauritz, *Vingarne* (1916).

Truffaut, François, *Les Quatre Cents Coups* (1959).

6 Disease, representation, and activism

Crossover: The Global Impact of AIDS (1988) and its reverberations

David Thorsén

Introduction

In the mid-1980s, HIV/AIDS was categorised by the World Health Organization (WHO) as one of the most significant global health crises that modern society had encountered. At the Fourth International AIDS Conference, in Stockholm in 1988, WHO's AIDS programme director, Dr Jonathan Mann, stated that the world had after an early phase of silence just entered the time of "global mobilisation against AIDS" (Mann 1988: 5). Today, decades into the pandemic, the global response to HIV and AIDS has been described as a mix of hope and gloom (Epstein 1996; Bayer and Oppenheimer 2000; Barnett and Whiteside 2006). The organisational responses to the multiple challenges of HIV and AIDS have, obviously, shifted not only over time but also within continents, nations, and communities. In Sweden, for example, NCA, the National Commission on AIDS ("Aidsdelegationen") was appointed by the government between 1985 and 1992 to coordinate the national response to the epidemic, an answer that included both new legislation and widespread information campaigns (Baldwin 2005; Thorsén 2005). Although significant in the late 1980s, the NAC was only one voice among others in the public discourse about HIV and AIDS in Sweden. During the last decades, numerous scholars have highlighted the need to examine not only how definitions of health and disease are articulated and negotiated – and more specifically, how governmental health promotion strategies are formulated and contested – but also to widen our analyses to new areas of society and social life, asking questions about, for example, how public health knowledge is produced, used, and transformed, and by whom, where, and why (Lemke 2011; Lupton 2003; Treichler 1999; Rose and Miller 1992).

In this chapter, I will analyse Staffan Hildebrand's film *Crossover: The Global Impact of AIDS* (1988) as a part of the intense debate on HIV and AIDS in late 1980s Sweden. Moreover, in a more explorative way, I will use *Crossover* as an example of how audio-visual media was used as a health promotion tool targeting the young. *Crossover*, produced to be broadcast on television and screened at particular information events in schools, had many supporters and was distributed widely all over the world. But *Crossover* also met with strong opposition, critics that saw the film as a provocative, redundant, and even

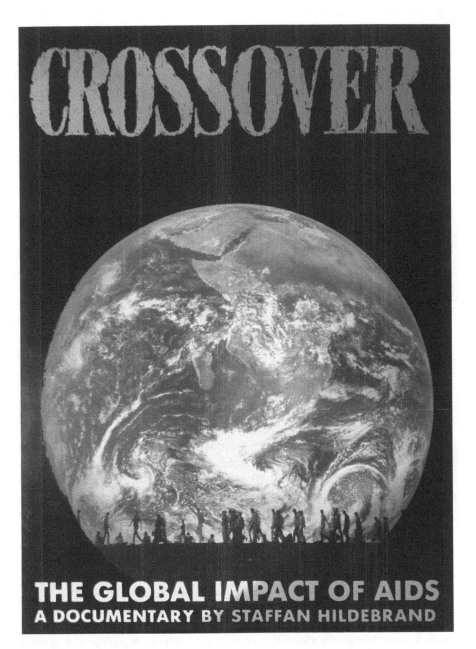

Figure 6.1 The poster for *Crossover*.

Source: Hildebrand, 1988.

ignorant statement about disease, sexual behaviour, norms, and identities. In the following, I will argue that *Crossover* is not only an example of how different meanings of HIV and AIDS were articulated – and disputed – in the late 1980s but also an instructive illustration of the importance both to acknowledge the variety of agents and activities present alongside governmental initiatives and to include a multiplicity of activities and audiences in the analysis of public health messages. As will be clear, it is not always easy to sort out different actors and their messages from each other. Therefore, my primary objectives are to present and analyse some aspects of the complex reception and reverberations of *Crossover* in a Swedish context and, by using *Crossover* as an example, to contribute to a discussion on the production and circulation of public health messages in the late twentieth century.

Crossover – production, distribution, and exhibition

As a nationally well-known journalist and filmmaker, Staffan Hildebrand had since the late 1970s produced a series of documentaries and information films but also some fiction films for movie theatres, starting with *G – som i gemenskap* ("C – as in community") from 1983. A unifying theme in most of the films from the 1980s, regardless of genre, is that they addressed various topics related to the experience of growing up: love and relations naturally, but also identity, drugs, violence, and the struggle to meet all the expectations and demands of grown-up society. To film critics, Hildebrand's filmmaking was often controversial, by some characterised as moralistic, plain, and oversimplified (*DN* 26 February, 1983). But, to many of the young, the films made an impression and were some-times, as *G*, commercial successes with large and enthralled audiences longing for the storyline, the music, the fashion, and the characters (*DN* 12 March 1983).

Hence it is not surprising that the press reported on Hildebrand as he in the summer of 1988 announced that he was making a film about HIV and AIDS and the global impact of the epidemic. "We have filmed in ten cities and on five con-tinents", Hildebrand told the major tabloid *Expressen* as he described the film and its international ambitions. "I have interviewed leading AIDS experts, police officers, prostitutes, dying AIDS patients, HIV-positives, priests, teen-agers and their worried mothers." In the article, Hildebrand states that he got the idea to do the film from his young audience, asking them what they wanted his next film to address. The framing of the article was sensationalist: "Glenn, 17, does anything for money. Hildebrand's AIDS film is shown throughout the world" ran the heading, illustrated by a large press photo from the film, depicting three Austral-ian boy prostitutes waiting for customers in the Sydney night. Furthermore, the participation of the American Hollywood actor Martin Sheen as the speaker voice was accentuated in the article. "Martin Sheen is my hero", Hildebrand explained, claiming that Sheen's participation had opened up new opportunities for the film's distribution and that Sheen personally contributed to the produc-tion economically by remitting his gauge. Financially, the film had been made possible by investments of a private production company as the NAC, according to Hildebrand, had turned him down owing to the high costs of the production (*Expressen* 8 June 1988).

The film was in many ways an international enterprise as it was produced by the production company Global Village and distributed by the Australian company Australian Beyond International. The journalist Lennart Alm, former information secretary in NAC, was one of the leading individuals behind the arrangement and Hildebrand himself was one of three private financiers (*Reporter* October 1988; *Landstingsfakta special* 2 June 1988).

Crossover was cut in at least two versions aimed to be shown to different audiences: one shorter version of approximately twenty-five minutes made for television, and one full version twice as long to be shown to live audiences followed by discussions. An early version of *Crossover* also served as the opening film at the Fourth International AIDS Conference, in Stockholm, 12–16 June 1988 (*Aftonbladet* 6 October 1988). But even though the conference was extensively covered by the Swedish press, no leading newspaper reported on the film or on its appearance in the opening ceremony (*DN* 12 June 1988; *SvD* 13 June 1988).

Things changed as the fifty-three-minute full version of *Crossover* was first screened publicly at a well-attended press conference in Stockholm, 5 October 1988. "Staffan Hildebrand's international documentary of AIDS is now finished", the national paper *Svenska Dagbladet* wrote the following day. The result was, according to the paper, a one-million-dollar film that reflected "the AIDS problem" on a global scale: from the tough street-life in the Bronx and child prostitution in Copacabana to young tourists in Paris, lorry-drivers in Uganda, female sex workers in the Philippines, patients at hospital wards in Australia, and "the gay men of San Francisco". Film – as a medium – was an exceptional and important tool to fight the epidemic, Hildebrand explained in the article. "Film enters the mind, combining your feelings with the intellectual. Film may change people's behaviour." And it was a "dramatic" and sometimes "upsetting" film that Hildebrand presented, *Svenska Dagbladet* reported in a short editorial comment the day after the press conference. *Crossover* was a dark film, the paper wrote, but not a film without hope. The future was represented by "the Enlighted youth", a new generation of informed and educated adolescents that had developed their own moral that differed "greatly from their parents' sex-liberal views" and for which a "condom and a permanent partner" was a matter of course (*SvD* 6 October 1988).

It is no surprise that *Svenska Dagbladet* and others focused on the different dimensions and morals of sexual behaviour addressed by the film. The necessity for a change in attitude towards sexual relations was obviously one of the main themes not only of *Crossover* but in the widely exposed – and at the time intensely discussed – official Swedish information campaigns (Henriksson 1988; Thorsén 2013). To the tabloid *Aftonbladet*, Hildebrand later explained that during the production he realised that the young people he interviewed for the film often shared a strong vision of a different world than the one they lived in that was shaped and ruled by their parents and their generation. "I've discovered among the young people around the world that they have the same moralism that

I have been criticized for in my movies", Hildebrand is quoted in the article as saying.

> They have no desire to take responsibility for what their parents caused. They do not want to live in a world of environmental pollution and sexual promiscuity. They want Amnesty, Greenpeace and profound love. There, I think, the young can educate their parents.
>
> (*Aftonbladet* 6 October 1988)

The narrative of *Crossover* is associative, relying more on moods and feelings than blank information. It is further built on the statements of Hildebrand's interviewees, leaving Martin Sheen's deep speaker voice to introduce, situate, and explain. At the end of *Crossover*, just to take one example, a young North American woman is interviewed sitting next to a young man in an inner-city park against a background of heavy skies and tall skyscrapers. Losing several friends to AIDS herself, she says she had noticed a change in attitude towards sex, especially among young people. "Not only because people are scared", she tells the interviewer, as the film moves to a scene where a young heterosexual couple are holding hands and kissing with the young woman's words as a voice-over. "But because they get so disillusioned with the whole lifestyle of promiscuity. They find that it is really empty. People now are looking for something deeper, something more real, something you can build on." The young woman's testimony is followed by a short scene where Professor Lars Olof Kallings – member of the NAC, chairman of the International AIDS Society, and the project's "scientific advisor", as he was presented in the press material – with his visual persona of the calm, grey-haired family doctor, addresses the young audience directly: "I would say to the young people, that you should not be afraid of sex and emotions. But use your head, use your mind to understand how the virus is spread, and protect yourself." *Crossover* ends with the words of Australian judge Michael D. Kirby, interviewed in a prominent library wearing his traditional black court dress. "It's really quite simple", he says as his words are accompanied by the images of a trendily dressed young heterosexual couple, hugging and kissing as they walk on the beach as the film fades out. "Until we have a cure and a vaccine, the only way we effectively can protect young people, is by the message of prevention" (*Crossover*, 1988, short version 25:45–26:40).

How the message of prevention was defined by *Crossover* and how it was received by different audiences will be discussed more in detail further on in this chapter. But, with regards to distribution, *Crossover* was an immediate success. The film was in a few months purchased by television companies in over thirty countries, including the American Discovery Channel (*Reporter* October 1988). In Sweden, a national tour in schools started in October 1988, reaching more than 20,000 high school students. The tour was composed as a two-and-a-half-hour package with the long version of the film, additional text materials (a teacher's guide for example), and an on-site discussion of the film by Hildebrand himself (*DN* 27 October 1988; *Aftonbladet* 2 December 1988). The version of

Crossover presented to the schools also began with a five-minute-long interview with Professor Lars Olof Kallings and Håkan Wrede, NAC's secretary, an addition accentuated in the official promotion material (*Aftonbladet* 2 December 1988). The demand for the film-and-discussion package was so massive that the City Council of Stockholm arranged an additional tour in the capital's local high schools in February and March 1989, reaching more than 22,000 students (*Kampen mot AIDS* 1989). At one occasion the tour was visited by the NAC chairman and minister of social affairs, Ms Gertrud Sigurdsen, an attendance reported in national papers (SvD 11 February, 1989).

The short version of *Crossover* also opened the National Swedish Broadcasting Cooperation's (SVT) full evening programme – "Together against AIDS" – on the first WHO-sponsored World AIDS Day, 1 December 1988. The film, now titled *Crossover: Världen efter AIDS* (*Crossover: The World After AIDS*), was introduced by one of the evening's hosts, Princess Christina of the royal family. The overall framing of *Crossover* both before and during the show was international, contemporary, young, and cool: it had a tempo as high as "an American newscast" and contained the "latest music", as *Svenska Dagbladet* wrote in an article promoting the film, and during the evening programme four young musicians from the Bronx appearing in the film performed live on stage. But, even if *Crossover* focused on a young audience – or maybe just because of that – some caution should be taken, *Svenska Dagbladet* continued. Several sequences in the film were described as "strong" and "emotional", especially Hildebrand's encounter with the Australian activist Lyle Taylor, in the paper presented as "a gay man lying on his death bed in a Sydney hospital". Hildebrand himself was also open-hearted about his own strong feelings, that the meeting had affected him deeply.

> I thought I was free of prejudice. But after all I learnt, I felt a screaming fear when I took his hand to say goodbye. How difficult is it for those who have no insight to give their full support to the AIDS victims?
> (*SvD* 1 December 1988; see also Hildebrand, *Expressen*, 27 November 1988)

Crossover – reception and criticism

Being broadcast on national Swedish television on World AIDS Day 1988, *Crossover* for the first time met a large and diverse nationwide audience. But *Crossover* had already provoked reactions and, sometimes, a strong criticism. In Stockholm City Council's newsletter about AIDS, for instance, *Crossover* was presented to the readers in September 1988. "It's an extraordinary achievement to produce such a highly qualified film production as *Crossover* in six months" (*Landstingsfakta special* 1 September 1988). In an article in *Aftonbladet*, Ann Colleen and Kjell Rindar from RFSL, Riksförbundet för sexuellt likaberättigande (the Swedish Federation for Lesbian, Bisexual, Transgender and Queer Rights), were more critical. On the positive side, *Crossover* openly promoted the use of condoms, something that Colleen and Rindar strongly supported, but the viewer was not given "a single relevant explanation of how to use a condom or any information on sexual techniques that are safe". And the message that it was dangerous to have many partners – "it is not if you practice safe sex", Colleen and Rindar stated forcefully – made some of the advice presented in the film hard for the audience to understand and even "irrelevant". Another problem was the film's attitude towards homosexuality, they continued. *Crossover* chiefly targeted young people but apparently only heterosexual youth, as the film's presentation of homosexuality – when it occurred – was "upsetting" and "offensive". The only gay people shown in the film were either boy prostitutes or middle-aged men dying in hospital beds, something that made the film both destructive and dangerous to a young homosexual audience as "positive identities" were "essential" to fight the spread of HIV. Colleen and Rindar concluded with a question: "Why, Staffan Hildebrand, is this group not given the same opportunity for identification and positive role models as the heterosexual youth?" (Colleen and Rindar 1988).

The gay magazine *Reporter* made a similar observation. Homosexual love was as absent in *Crossover* as beautiful heterosexual couples were "plentiful", the magazine concluded in a full-page article on the film in October 1988. Interviewed for the article, Hildebrand, perhaps unexpectedly in the light of earlier statements, seemed to agree with the reporter. It was a "mistake", he said, that the film did not pay more attention to homosexuality in general and young gay men in particular:

> It's a big misstep that we don't have male couples hugging and kissing in the film.... If we would have had 20 minutes of boys doing just that, it would have worked out nicely in the picture and be pleasant to watch too.
>
> (*Reporter* October 1988)

The interview in *Reporter* did not stop a growing discussion about *Crossover* and the film's – according to its critics – moralistic overtones and negative representation of homosexuality. For example, during the autumn of 1988 one RFSL activist invited himself to accompany the school tour to, as it was described in *Reporter*, "balance the negative content" of the film and present himself as an "example" of a proud young gay man (*Reporter* January 1989).

Individuals were not the only ones to openly criticise *Crossover*. The day after the film was broadcast on Swedish television, the tone was coarse, even hostile. In the leading national newspaper *Dagens Nyheter*, Katarina Lindahl from RFSU (Riksförbundet för sexuell upplysning) said that *Crossover* was a film that "drives prejudice". According to Lindahl, the film neither increased people's knowledge nor provided them with tools or power to fight HIV and AIDS. The result was almost the opposite: being "so seductive" and communicating a "feeling of dread", the message of the film was that "ordinary women suffer while homosexuals are punished for their sins". The official City Council AIDS organisation of Stockholm, LAFA (Landstinget förebygger AIDS), was just as critical, also disassociating themselves from the film. "We do not want this film", Anders Bohlin, project manager of LAFA, told the paper. But it was not just the film that did not meet his organisation's expectations, he continued. The whole extensive communication programme built around the film – foremost the local school tours – was simply not an effective way to address such a complex issue as HIV and AIDS. Instead, Bohlin argued, it would be much more efficient to rely on educators at the local level, teachers and other professionals within the schools, and to trust their competence to meet their students' needs and questions. Bohlin's sharp criticism was thus not directed merely at the film itself. From his perspective, *Crossover* had become an unwelcome and insufficient part of the local health promotion strategy, and by that an opposing activity to the responsibilities and expertise of his own organisation and other important agents on the local level. In an official comment, Georg Sved from RFSL Stockholm was even harsher. According to Sved, *Crossover* was nothing less than a disaster. "The film erodes the opportunities for the people who want to make a difference", he told *Dagens Nyheter*. "The film offers no future for young gay men" (*DN* 2 December 1988).

Crossover was not the first of Hildebrand's films to be denounced. As a tool to highlight complicated issues to a young audience, the usage of Hildebrand's films was already a controversial method, especially when practised in schools, where the combination of film and discussion was often conducted in the school auditorium and attendance was mandatory. The decision, for example, to show Hildebrand's film *Stockholmsnatt* ("Stockholm Night") from 1987 addressing the problem of youth violence – a tour that reached up to one million students nationwide – was condemned by many, not at least several teachers (*DN* 19 May, 1987).

At the same time, it is noticeable that most of the contemporary critics did not have any major objectives to the medical content in *Crossover*; it was the film's "attitude", as *Dagens Nyheter* put it, that provoked all the strong words and disapproval. Staffan Hildebrand was also given an opportunity to respond to his critics directly. "Those who attack my movies are always the same people," he defended himself. "It is the cultural establishment which is based on the revolution of the 1960s when norms and morals were demolished". *Crossover* should instead be seen as a film made directly for the young, a film based on "my personal position and my own experiences", he continued:

AIDS is for me a way of looking at the world as an artist. It is a film based on the same personal perceptions I have about drugs and violence. I have worked in the same way as in my previous feature films and documentaries.

But even as Hildebrand strongly refuted his critics, he did not deny that *Crossover* was a film driven by a strong personal ethos. To those who claimed that *Crossover* was full of prejudice – about sexuality in general but homosexuality in particular – he tried to clarify his mission by explaining that his own ideas and values of sex and relations converged with what he saw in the upcoming generation.

"Youngsters of today long for romance and a message of faithfulness and love", he stated.

> I want to go against the current, against the commercialism of society, against the liberal mass media that say: Try everything! I want to get back to the spirit of the post-war years and give standards of sex and drugs.
>
> (*DN* 2 December 1988)

A strong personal opinion in complex topics – especially concerning sex, drugs, and violence – is something that is evident not only in *Crossover* but in the general production by Hildebrand during the 1980s. The reception of *Crossover* is therefore no exception and Hildebrand's answer was more or less the same as to the critics of his other films. "A movie can be made in many ways but no way fits everyone", he says about *Crossover* in February 1989, for example. "I make movies in my own way and for schoolchildren. And I accompany the movies to discuss the questions that arise" (*Kampen mot AIDS* 1989: 6–9). *Crossover* is hence one of several examples of what Hildebrand, at various occasions and in other films like *Ingen kan älska som vi. En kärleksfilm av Staffan Hildebrand* ("Nobody Can Love as We Do. A Love Movie by Staffan Hildebrand"), also from 1988, communicated as a generation-specific shift in values: away from what he described as a pleasure-seeking and self-centred legacy of the late 1960s, to a new kind of emotional profoundness, a change to the sincere or a genuine from-the-heart position concerning sex and sexual relations. And, interestingly, the message of an ongoing shift was in Hildebrand's rhetoric, combined with both an overt national nostalgia of a lost world – the positive, collective, secure, and conscientious world of the expanding Swedish welfare state, the *folkhem* – and with an intrinsic sensitivity to contemporary urban youth culture, to the newest music, fashion, international influences and trends (*SvD* 4 September 1988. Svensk Filmdatabas, 1988).

The impression of Hildebrand's mission is therefore somewhat ambivalent, an entangled combination of old and new. The various cinematic expressions of *Crossover* – the photo, the music, and the tempo of the film – clearly conversed with the ambition to reach a particular kind of audience: the young. But, on the other hand, the criticism of *Crossover* was not primarily focused on the films audio-visual configuration but on its message and, even more importantly, what consequences – the effect – that the presented message was expected to have on its audience. The knowledge *Crossover* communicated was not only contested by various critics among its audiences; the film was also immediately incorporated into a wider contemporaneous discussion about identity and sexuality, drugs and inequality, globalisation and the future.

Crossover – activist and academic responses

Soon after *Crossover*, in 1989, Hildebrand made a second film about HIV and AIDS produced by Global Village, the film *At Risk*. *At Risk* served as the opening film of the International AIDS Conference in Montreal in 1989 but Hildebrand also, now in partnership with and sponsored by the National Board of Health (Socialstyrelsen), did a tour with the film in schools in eleven Swedish cities (*Aftonbladet* 23 January, 1990). *At Risk* covered in parts the same themes and had the same international focus as *Crossover* but presented, for example, a bisexual leading character and was also produced as a mix of documentary and fiction, for instance using dramatised scenes driving the narrative forward. The film, just as *Crossover*, came in different versions at different length for different audiences but the criticisms, not least from gay activists, was still harsh. For example, in the summer of 1989 RFSL nominated – and awarded – Hildebrand to the organisation's yearly "Homophobia Price", an award that wanted to pay attention to someone that, according to RFSL, had made "serious violations during the year by nurturing prejudice about homosexuals". RFSL motivated its choice by saying that *Crossover* and *At Risk* presented a "hostile message" and "portrayed homosexuality in a negative and repulsive way". Hildebrand himself had also, according to RFSL, an "outstanding ability to be silent about homosexuality in his films about AIDS" (*SvD* 13 August, 1989).

RFSL's attention to *Crossover* shows that the debate about the film was still active in 1989, one year after its premiere. The most substantial analysis of *Crossover* was also presented during that time, an analysis by the British scholar and photographer Simon Watney. In the premiere issue of the first academic journal on homosexuality in Sweden, *Lambda nordica – populärvetenskaplig tidskrift om homosexualitet*, edited by the social scientist Benny Henriksson and published in March 1989, Watney made a comprehensive – and very critical – review of *Crossover*. But Watney's review must be understood as something more than yet another critical remark on *Crossover*. Watney's article is one of few examples in Swedish of what Deborah Lupton later defined as "the politics of representation", an analysis or a cultural activity that has both political objectives and a clear vision of the political effects of its arguments and expressions. Or, as Lupton puts it, "The potential to resist oppressive and stigmatizing discourses and practices is liberated and artistic or cultural criticism endeavours become activism" (Lupton 2003: 83).

In his article, Watney addresses many aspects of *Crossover* to explore – in his eyes – the film's many weaknesses, errors and dangers. One of the things Watney discusses is fear. Fear runs like a "subtle allusion" throughout the film, he argues, and manifests in the dialogue and in the choice of experts, places, and situations visited. In *Crossover*, the director's own fear is amplified and transferred to the audience. "With the importance of television in our modern world", Watney writes, "and the vital need to produce effective information on AIDS, we need to consider *Crossover* very threatening, especially if we take into account the audience for which it is intended, namely the younger generation" (Watney 1989: 207, my translation).

Another theme addressed by Watney is how *Crossover* combines AIDS with drugs, criminality, and poverty. The socially devastated and deserted neighbourhoods of the Bronx are "the perfect environment for the virus to thrive", Sheen's speaker voice states, leaving one out of sixteen inhabitants infected with the virus (*Crossover*, 1988, short version, 11:50–11:53). In a Swedish context, AIDS had an exceptionally strong – but complex – connection to drugs and drug abuse. Drugs was one of the major political issues at the time and many of the official governmental actions – including legal possibilities to detain individuals at special hospital wards – was in both argument and practice connected to drug users (Thorsén 2013; 2005; Vallgårda 2007). The emphasis on drugs and poverty in *Crossover* had therefore a potentially two-way outcome on the Swedish audience: on the one hand, that the connection between drugs and HIV was further strengthened and, on the other hand, as Watney also states explicitly, that HIV "implies little or no threat to young white Swedes" (Watney 1989: 201, my translation).

The global aspects of HIV and AIDS in *Crossover* were, according to Watney, based on a misunderstanding of the epidemiology of the virus. *Crossover* was an example of what Watney called "AIDS Safari" journalism.

> We are transported to a lot of exotic places all around the world, from Manilla to the Bronx. Still, the impression is always the same. Movies like this are based on the deeply misleading assumption that we could and should consider AIDS as a global phenomenon rather than a series of separate epidemics, affecting different societies and cultures in different ways.
>
> (Watney 1989: 207–208, my translation)

AIDS was better understood as a pandemic consisting of many different epidemics, Watney argued. And, instead of being able to learn from each other, from how HIV/AIDS was handled in different countries and communities, the viewer of *Crossover* was left in intellectual, emotional and moral despair.

> Like safari travellers of former times, he [Hildebrand] has brought home the cinematic equivalent to the worn zebra-skin and silk bales, plus a lot of glamorous and misleading conceptions that teach us nothing about the communities they claim to represent.
>
> (Watney 1989: 208, my translation)

Watney here converges some of the arguments about AIDS that just had started to be formulated, analyses that developed in more detail and force in the years to come (Treichler 1999; Farmer 1992). But, in a Swedish context, *Crossover* communicates an understanding of the epidemic that in many ways reinforced an already widespread idea that the situation in other countries was not only separated from the Swedish epidemic – leaving the rest of the world unsafe and going abroad even more hazardous – but also that the development in countries more affected was a horrifying indication of what awaited Sweden unless sufficient measures were taken (Thorsén 2013; 2005; Bredström 2008). Even the name of the film resembled some of that anxiety: the crossover, the passage of boundaries and borders, the threat to us from them. "*Crossover* takes its name from the situation in Sydney, Australia", Watney unfolded his argument. "Rather than displaying gay men as the most threatened by the infection, they are depicted as the threat" (Watney 1989: 214, my translation).

And, being a film for the young, the generation that will be shaping the future, *Crossover* is a wreckage, Watney ends his article.

> Like the National Commission on AIDS, the people behind *Crossover* seem to have learned little or none from those who have the major experience of AIDS.... To me, it seems like a waste of a lot of money making *Crossover*, a film that will only serve to reinforce ignorance and prejudice. It is a very sad reflection of the Swedish AIDS policy that a movie like this would come after *eight years* of the epidemic. It is even more regrettable that the film is shown in schools for young people who have little access to other, more reliable and helpful information.... The young of Sweden deserve better. One day they will get up and demand it. And that day cannot come fast enough.
>
> (Watney 1989: 217, my translation)

For Watney, *Crossover* was not only insidious in its description of homosexuality; it was also severely simplifying the social, political, and moral aspects of the epidemic. The film was not only inadequate when it came to the information or knowledge it communicated; it was also – as a cinematic representation of AIDS and its global impact – in itself a dangerous argument with potentially devastating effects. Watney's criticism of *Crossover* is therefore an analogy to Douglas Crimp's contemporaneous but much more cited analysis of the photographer Nicholas Nixon's exhibition "Pictures of People" displayed at the Museum of Modern Art in New York in 1988. The exhibition at MOMA was dominated by large photographs of predominantly young males devastated by the disease, often portrayed laying passively in a bed. "Certainly", Crimp argues, "we can say that these representations do not help us ... because the best they can do is elicit pity, and pity is not solidarity". For Crimp, it is therefore important to increase an awareness that representations of AIDS are effective epistemological and political tools. "We must continue to demand and create our own counter images", he concludes:

> But we must also recognize that every image of a PWA [person with AIDS] is a *representation*, and formulate our activist demands not in relation to the 'truth' of the image, but in relation to the conditions of its construction and to its social effects.
>
> (Crimp 2002 [1988]: 100)

Conclusion

Audio-visual representations – like Staffan Hildebrand's *Crossover: The Global Impact of AIDS*, from 1988 – are important in shaping our understanding of health and illness. As shown above, *Crossover* is an example of how a film can be understood not only to possess an ability to contribute to its audience's understanding of HIV and AIDS but also that this knowledge could – and often is – challenged by its audiences. Furthermore, *Crossover* demonstrates how difficult it is to draw clear boundaries between different actors in the formulation of specific health messages and strategies of health promotion. There is, for example, an ambiguity regarding both the production and distribution of *Crossover* concerning who the key players were and what their significance was. The links between the NCA, other public bodies and authorities – not least various agents within the County Council of Stockholm – and the film are in practice both hard to determine and sometimes contradictory. *Crossover* was not financed directly by the NCA or by any Swedish governmental agency, yet central actors behind the film's production team were closely linked to NCA and individuals involved – and appearing – in the film were representatives of the NCA. The local and national distribution of *Crossover* was clearly made with the help of municipal organisations or City Councils. Even at the level of exhibition, which was predominantly carried out in public places such as schools and communal youth clubs and financed by the local authorities, leading national representatives officially endorsed and legitimated the film and its display. Even if it is obvious that *Crossover* was not formally a part of the national Swedish AIDS information campaign, *Crossover* still existed in a kind of symbolic symbiosis with other publicly sanctioned statements in the national AIDS discourse.

Over time, Hildebrand has in many ways modified his understanding of HIV and AIDS since the late 1980s. But *Crossover* is, as has been shown in this chapter, the troublesome start of a longer commitment that later came to be the Face of AIDS film archive. Therefore, the reverberations of *Crossover* – both as a historical artefact and an ongoing ambition – are still heard in our time.

References

Aftonbladet (1988). "Hildebrands film om aids", 6 October.
Aftonbladet (1988). "Här är rapparna från Bronx som överraskade i TV-galan", 2 December.
Aftonbladet (1990). "Att gilla killar är inte så märkvärdigt", 23 January.
Baldwin, Peter (2005). *Disease and Democracy. The State Faces AIDS in the Industrialized World*. Berkeley, CA: University of California Press.
Barnett, Tony and Alan Whiteside (2006). *AIDS in the Twenty-First Century. Disease and Globalization*. Fully revised and updated ed. London: Palgrave Macmillan.
Bayer, Ronald and Gerhald M. Oppenheimer (2000). *AIDS Doctors. Voices from the Epidemic: An Oral History*. Oxford and New York: Oxford University Press.
Bredström, Anna (2008). *Safe Sex, Unsafe Identities: Intersections of "Race", Gender and Sexuality in Swedish HIV/AIDS Policy*. Linköping: Linköping University.
Colleen, A. and R. Rindar (1988). "Får inte bögar vara så lyckliga". *Aftonbladet*, 27 October.
Crimp, Douglas (2002 [1988]). "Portraits of people with AIDS". Reprinted in *Melancholia and Moralism. Essays on AIDS and Queer Politics*. Cambridge, MA: MIT Press.

Dagens Nyheter (1983). "Sörgårgshistoria inom ram av betong", 26 February.
Dagens Nyheter (1983). "Samtal om 'G'. Allt måste inga va' verklighet", 12 March.
Dagens Nyheter (1987). "En miljon ungdomar ser Stockholsnatt", 19 May.
Dagens Nyheter (1988). "Trots flera framsteg. Inget vaccin för aids i sikte ännu", 12 June.
Dagens Nyheter (1988). "Landstinget bekostar turné", 27 October.
Dagens Nyheter (1988). "Helkväll om kampen mot aids", 1 December.
Dagens Nyheter (1988). "Hildebrands film får stark kritik", 2 December.
Epstein, Steven (1996). *Impure Science: AIDS, Activism, and the Politics of Knowledge.* Berkeley, CA: University of California Press.
Expressen (1988). "Glenn, 17, gör allt för pengar. Hildebrands aidsfilm visas i hela världen", 8 June.
Farmer, Paul (1992). *AIDS and Accusation. Haiti and the Geography of Blame.* Berkeley, CA: University of California Press.
Henriksson, Benny (1988). *Social Democracy and Societal Control. A Critical Analysis of Swedish AIDS Policy.* Stockholm: Institutet för sociala studier.
Hildebrand, Staffan (1988). "Döden är här – och överallt. Pojken säger ja till smittan", *Aftonbladet*, 28 November.
Kampen mot AIDS (1989). "Staffan Hildebrand på turné med Crossover", 1: 6–9.
Landstingsfakta special (1988). "Crossover. En dokumentärfilm av världsformat", 2 June.
Landstingsfakta special (1988). "Cross-over. Skakande AIDS-dokumentär", 1 September.
Lemke, Thomas (2011). *Foucault, Governmentality, and Critique.* Boulder, CO: Paradigm.
Lupton, Deborah (2003). *Medicine as Culture.* 2nd ed. London: SAGE.
Mann, Jonathan M. (1988). "The Global Picture of AIDS", address presented at the fourth International AIDS Conference, Stockholm, Sweden, 12 June 1988, http://apps.who.int/iris/bitstream/10665/60110/1/WHO_GPA_DIR_88.2.pdf.
Reporter (1988). "Staffan Hildebrand om sin aidsfilm. 'Bara heteropussar en miss…'", 10 (October).
Reporter (1989). "1988", 1 (January).
Rose, Nikolas and Peter Miller (1992). "Political Power beyond the State. Problems in Government", *The British Journal of Sociology*, 43(2): 173–205.
Svensk filmdatabas (1988). Ingen kan älska som vi. En kärleksfilm av Staffan Hildebrand, www.sfi.se/sv/svensk-filmdatabas/Item/?itemid=15956&type=MOVIE&iv=Comments.
Svenska Dagbladet (1988). "Jag vill få igång en dialog", 4 September.
Svenska Dagbladet (1988). "Aidsfilm som kan ge unga nytt hopp", 6 October.
Svenska Dagbladet (1988). "Dystra siffror på Stocholmskonferensen: En miljon aidsfall om fem år", 13 June.
Svenska Dagbladet (1988). "En känsloladdad aidsdokumentär", 1 December.
Svenska Dagbladet (1989). "'Tillsammans är vi oemotståndliga'", 13 August.
Svenska Dagbladet (1989). "Sigurdsens nya roll: Aidskampen huvudsaken", 11 February.
Thorsén, David (2005). "Epidemic Times. A Brief History of HIV/AIDS in Sweden", in M-L. Foller and H. Thörn (eds), *No Name Fever: AIDS in the Age of Globalisation.* Lund: Studentlitteratur.
Thorsén, David (2013). *Den svenska aidsepidemin. Ankomst, bemötande, innebörd.* Acta Universitatis Upsaliensis. Uppsala Studies in History of Ideas 44. Uppsala: Uppsala University.
Treichler, Paula A. (1999). *How to Have Theory in an Epidemic. Cultural Chronicles of AIDS.* Durham, NC, and London: Duke University Press.
Vallgårda, Signild (2007). "Problematizations and Path Dependency. HIV/AIDS Policies in Denmark and Sweden", *Medical History*, 51: 99–112.

Watney, Simon (1989). "Crossover. En film av Staffan Hildebrand", *Lambda nordica*, 1: 206–217.

Films and TV productions

Hildebrand, Staffan, *G – som i gemenskap* (1983).
Hildebrand, Staffan, *Stockholmsnatt* (1987).
Hildebrand, Staffan, *Crossover: The Global Impact of AIDS* (1988).
Hildebrand, Staffan, *Ingen kan älska som vi. En kärleksfilm av Staffan Hildebrand* (1988).
Hildebrand, Staffan, *At Risk* (1989).

7 A positive positive?

Intersectional analysis of identification and counter-identification in three contemporary HIV narratives

Desireé Ljungcrantz

Who are we, the people portrayed as having our faces linked to HIV? Who do we appear to be and what does that do to the cultural imaginaries of HIV? As a person who has had HIV for approximately fifteen years, I have certain experiences of it. As a person born in Sweden, with light-coloured skin and Swedish as my mother tongue, as a person who might be read as heterosexual and a rather feminine woman, I have some privileges that affect my opportunities to negotiate HIV and the cultural imaginaries surrounding and shaping it. I will give an example from a few years ago, when the Public Health Agency of Sweden approached me with a request to be a poster girl for the campaign "HIV is not what it used to be":

> I am supposed to be one of four examples of how it could be to have HIV in contemporary Sweden. Should I be a role model? It brings me back to things that people have said to me over the years; that I would be a good representative for HIV because I am "a sort of cute girl" or that I "seem to be a happy person for whom things have worked out." I laugh. I should probably work as an example that "anyone" could have HIV and that life can still be good. Despite HIV…. I phone them a couple of days later and say that I am pleased about the inquiry and that I can imagine participating if I can be a researcher with HIV. They say no.
> (Auto-fictive notes, originally published in Swedish in Ljungcrantz 2017)

Representing HIV in the public sphere is an important part of transforming the negative cultural imaginaries surrounding it. Questions about which persons are represented and in what ways are important in order to make room for the diverse ways of having and experiencing HIV. In this chapter, I will explore the portrayal of HIV-positivity and the phenomenon of HIV in a contemporary Swedish context, focusing on the documentary *The Longest Journey Is the Journey Within – The Film about Steve* (*Den längsta resan, är resan inåt*, Hildebrand 2015), which is available on various sites online, about Steve Sjöquist, an HIV-positive activist.[1]

The analysis will be intersectional, exploring identifications and counter-identifications of an HIV-positive person. Identification means an identity that is based on the affirmation of "I am", including different identity characteristics that relate to social categorisations. Counter-identifications are in line with "I am not" statements, where the identity is built upon oppositions to other identity characteristics or social categorisations (Muñoz 1999; Fuss 1995). Identities might be multiple, resulting in the need to use the plural-form identifications rather than identification in singular form. Identifications are more internal than external in this text, hence the statements and positions made by the main characters. I will also analyse the dramaturgical formation through these HIV narratives and how the dramaturgical curve shapes the HIV-positive self.

When exploring representations of HIV in popular culture the ideas of HIV in the surrounding society are an important part of the context and understanding of HIV. The cultural imaginaries, i.e. ideas and images about a phenomenon (Dawson 1994), in this chapter of HIV in Sweden, are related to a distance from HIV where HIV belongs to other places and other people, as well as a distance from people who by the majoritarian society might be expected to have HIV or be regarded as deviant in other ways, i.e. homosexual people, drug users, sex workers, or immigrants (see e.g. Nilsson Schönnesson 2001; Johannisson 2002; Bredström 2008; Rydström 2008; Thorsén 2013). Previous research has shown that the discursive understanding of HIV and AIDS has been interconnected with moralistic, homophobic and racist connotations (see e.g. Bredström 2008; Johannisson 2002; Svensson 2013; Thorsén 2013; see also Treichler 1999; Patton 1990) as well as fear and shame, often defined as HIV stigma, which makes HIV a lonely illness to live with (see e.g. Eriksson 2012; Lindberg, Wettergren, Wiklander, Svedhem-Johansson and Eriksson 2014; Ljungcrantz 2017; the Public Health Agency of Sweden 2013; Rydström 2015).

In Sweden, HIV can be described as a minoritarian position and experience, affecting approximately 7,000 people. Worldwide, approximately 36.9 million people have an HIV diagnosis (UNAIDS 2015; The Public Health Agency of Sweden 2016). The phenomenon of HIV in Sweden can be contextualised in relation to three circumstances: First, medical care and HIV medications are free of charge and accessible. Second, HIV is regulated by the Contagious Disease Act (SFS 2004:168), according to which medical doctors working with HIV patients act as both caregivers and legislative controllers. Third, there is an information duty laid out in the Contagious Disease Act (SFS 2004:168) whereby people who have HIV must inform a potential partner before having sex. Failure to do so is criminalised and regulated under the Penal Code (SFS 162: 700) as physical assault, and an option exists for medical institutions to isolate a person who does not follow the law (The Public Health Agency of Sweden and the National Board of Health and Welfare 2010; UNAIDS 2016; Weait 2011; The Disease Act 2016). However, in November 2013, the information duty was revised so that a so-called HIV patient who is taking HIV medication on a regular basis, has a very low virus level and uses a condom while having sex can negotiate with their medical doctor to dispense with the information duty before having sex. This implies that the frameworks for living with HIV in Sweden are undergoing negotiations.

This chapter begins with a part describing the empirical material, methodology and theoretical framework, followed by an analytical part divided into three sections. The first section focuses on medical progress and the desire to be healed. The second section explores identifications and the tendency to individualise the disease and to frame lust for life as making the difference between surviving and dying of the disease. In the third section, I analyse counter-identifications in the formation of HIV-positivity and discuss some missing links in the documentary. However, it should be remembered that the documentary is short and is a very small selection from the Face of AIDS film archive. I conclude by discussing normalisation strategies and the risk of creating borders and divisions between respectable and disreputable HIV positives.

Material, method and theoretical framework

The empirical material analysed in this chapter is, as stated, the short documentary film *The Longest Journey Is the Journey Within*, featuring the protagonist Steve Sjöquist. The material is a 68:34-minute long documentary film, available online, and is a part of the Face of AIDS film archive. In contrast to most of the archive material, this film is fully accessible online. The film contains moving images, speech and text. I will focus on all these dimensions in the film. I will also make some comparisons with other HIV narratives: the autobiographies *Ophelias resa* ("Ophelia's Journey", Larsson and Haanyama Ørum 2007) and *Mitt positiva liv* ("My Positive Life", Lundstedt and Blankens 2012). Consequently, the principal characters in this text will be Steve, Ophelia and Andreas, the protagonist of *Mitt positiva liv*. These three sets of material are examples of contemporary biographical accounts of HIV. The film was transcribed by the author of this chapter in order to be able to include quotes. The film is in Swedish with English subtitles, the autobiographies are in Swedish and the translation of all quotes was also performed by the author.

The method used is a critical reading and thematic analysis of the documentary, making a norm-critical and intersectional analysis with the aim of identifying tendencies and patterns that are important for understanding both the normalising strategies that people use when portraying HIV and the ongoing transformation of cultural imaginaries of the disease in a contemporary Swedish context.

Theoretically, the analysis is based on the understanding that how a phenomenon is portrayed both describes how that phenomenon is understood in that context *and* shapes the phenomenon (Butler 1997). How HIV is represented in the public sphere is therefore significant in the meaning-making processes of HIV. The central questions that the chapter aims to answer are: How are HIV and "the HIV-positive self" narrated and imagined? And how are normativities and deviations negotiated and narrated? The analysis of the documentary will be performed through theoretical conversations with intersectional perspectives on identities, normativities and deviation (see e.g. Fuss 1995; Butler 1997; Muñoz 1999; Lykke 2010).

Intersectional approaches focus on normativities and hierarchies and the processes by which these aspects are negotiated. By normativities, in this text I particularly mean norms that are connected to heteronormativity, i.e. promoting mono-normative, monogamous coupledom and family-centred ways to live in pairs that are regarded as respectable in both sexual and gender terms (see e.g. Rubin 1984; Butler 1990; Berlant and Warner 1998; Skeggs 1997; Edelman 2004; Halberstam 2005; Roseneil 2006; Gustavson 2006; Kean 2015). Deviations from these norms could be classified as promiscuous. Respectability can be regarded as a locus for normative lines (see e.g. Butler 1997; Skeggs 1997; Ahmed 2006; Bremer 2011; Ljungcrantz 2017), along which a person, a body and a life are regarded as respectable, liveable and acceptable. Respectability also relates to norms around health, with an HIV-negative status as a precondition (McRuer 2006) and Swedishness and whiteness as interrelated categories that create lines of exclusion and inclusion (Mattsson 2005; Hübinette and Lundström 2011). These normative lines are negotiated in and are a part of the phenomenon of HIV, especially since the cultural imaginaries on HIV are historically charged (Johannisson 2002; Svensson 2013; Thorsén 2013; see also Patton 1990; Treichler 1999).

The chapter also focuses on the documentary as a chronic illness narrative. Some AIDS narratives portray people dying of AIDS-related conditions, while others portray people surviving the disease (see e.g. Kleinman 1988; Frank 1995; Couser 1997; 2010; Lupton 2003; Jurecic 2012). *The Longest Journey Is the Journey Within – The Film about Steve* is, however, not primarily and only an AIDS narrative but a retrospective AIDS narrative and a survivor narrative transforming into an HIV narrative. With HIV narrative, I mean a story about living with HIV as a chronic illness. Hence, the chapter explores the genre of contemporary HIV narratives as it emerges from AIDS narratives through pharmaceutical progress.

Another aspect to consider is that disease narratives and illness narratives have a history of being often separated, that is, as narratives about either the physical or the social dimensions of, for example, a diagnosis. Artur Frank (1995) argues that this distinction is too strict, in that HIV as a phenomenon might be regarded as both physical and social. Nevertheless, it is the social, cultural aspect of HIV that is the focus of this text. HIV narratives can function as a case study for illness narratives, i.e. novels and autobiographical accounts of living with an illness, in contrast to the disease understood as the medical aspects of an illness (Kleinman 1988). Writing and reading illness narratives might be a way to "heal" through understanding and reorienting in a new situation (Frank 1995: 182). In this case, the narratives are about the chronic medical state of HIV and analysing them might be a way of understanding the meaning-making processes of HIV today.

Identifications: medical progress, the desire to heal

The Longest Journey Is the Journey Within – The Film about Steve starts at the World AIDS Conference in 2013, where Steve Sjöquist, the protagonist of the story, is filmed and asked questions by the filmmaker, Staffan Hildebrand, who is behind the camera. Hildebrand asks: "It's been 25 years since you got your diagnosis. How are today's AIDS conferences different?" Steve answers:

It's mostly that it isn't a sense of hopelessness anymore. People have always been committed, and even during the tough years when people died, and it was very … there was a lot of focus on death and memorial services. That was rough. Today, the feeling is a lot more hopeful. There are a lot of different treatments, and people here lobby hard for access, that these treatments should be available to anyone who needs them. There's a lot of hope now, and the focus is on when we're going to solve this. It's amazing to feel that, being here. Especially in my case.

The film portrays a survivor from the 1980s and 1990s, a senior HIV-positive person with life experiences that parallel medical developments. Steve works as an example of an individual carrier of the medical genealogies of HIV and AIDS, on which the film focuses. In this story of the history of HIV in Sweden, hope and the expectation of finding a cure and "ending AIDS" are argued for. There is a tendency in the story to construct a binary between then and now, death and life, suffering and hope rather than discontinuities.

Another scene in which this can be observed is when Steve and the medical doctor Per Hedman are interviewed about the 1990s. The encounter is emotional, with the medical doctor being asked to describe the situation for Steve. The conversation ends by discussing Steve's luck timewise, since 1996 was the year when the combination treatment, ART, the first effective HIV medication, became available. Hedman explains:

Because of your will to live and because of our medication, you made it into 1997. And then you recovered, and you've soldiered on ever since.

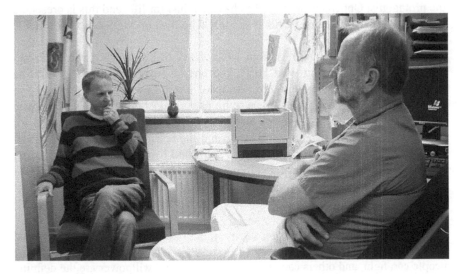

Figure 7.1 Steve and his physician. *The Longest Journey Is the Journey Within.*
Source: Hildebrand 2015.

This statement reflects how the film is set in a society dominated by neo-liberalism and wellness syndrome. By neo-liberalism, I mean the dominant ideology that is market-driven and claims that choice is equivalent to individual agency (Connell 2010; Luxton 2010). The wellness syndrome refers to the idea that individuals are expected to improve themselves both physically and mentally. A part of this framework is to regard disease and illness as a failure of the individual's attitude, according to Barbara Ehrenreich (2009), who argues that this discourse presumes that an attitude that is not good enough causes death to occur more easily (Ehrenreich 2009; Cederström and Spicer 2015). Within this individualist, neo-liberal context, suffering is not understood as an acceptable part of life but as something that hinders happiness and must be conquered (Cederström and Spicer 2015; Svenaeus 2013).

Identifications: alive and positive

In the documentary, the protagonist is portrayed as a person with a strong will who, assisted by a stroke of luck in terms of when effective medications were introduced, survived because of that will. The protagonist is represented as a strong hero, in line with survivor narratives of putting up a fight against disease (see e.g. Frank 1995; Kleinman 1988; Lupton 2003; Jurecic 2012) and with the wellness discourse (Ehrenreich 2009; Cederström and Spicer 2015). Steve is portrayed as a physical and emotional survivor and can be categorised as a white, middle-aged man, homosexual and a part of the Pride movement, an HIV activist and a Christian deacon, calm and respectable.

The quote above from *The Longest Journey Is the Journey Within – The Film about Steve*, relates to a passage in the autobiography *Ophelias resa*, in which the protagonist Ophelia is portrayed as having a lust for life, and this is presented as the difference between her and the people who died of AIDS-related illnesses:

> She remembers her friends from Noah's Ark [a Swedish support organisation for people living with HIV], the ones who regained their lives. She thinks about the ones who did not make it. On how much the will to live mattered, how strong it had to be to hit back against the virus. The ones who did not manage and gave in, they hadn't survived.... Nobody knows for how long the medications will work and the resistance progress. However, Ophelia is a survivor. To never give up, and to manage a little bit more, despite the exclusion and side effects – that is the feeling that she would like to describe when she is giving lectures about her illness.
>
> (Larsson and Haanyama Ørum 2007: 271–272)

Ophelia is portrayed as a strong survivor, in contrast to other people who died of AIDS-related diseases. This way of portraying HIV, as something that some people can fight, and others cannot, where strength and willpower are the defining qualities, tends to individualise and psychologise an illness or a disease (also see Ljungcrantz 2017). This kind of victim blaming reproduces a cultural imaginary of an opposition between fighters and losers, hence making room and acceptance for certain kinds of experiences and people, excluding others.

Similar descriptions are found in *Mitt positiva liv*. Here, Andreas is portrayed as identifying with health and happiness, which stand in binary opposition to AIDS and HIV, which are related to filth, death and victims.

> It was just so hard to regard myself as HIV infected. It felt so dirty. So sullied and shitty. And I was far from dirty. That super social, lovely and funny guy. The one who was always laughing. That was me. That was my image of myself, and it had absolutely nothing to do with an emaciated old AIDS victim. I could not be both, so I had to choose, and the choice was easy. I would continue to be my healthy self, for that was how I felt. It did not hurt anywhere. My eyesight was perfect and my teeth sat where they should. HIV-Andreas had to hide and pretend he did not exist.
>
> (Lundstedt and Blankens 2012: 96)

This quote contains both identificatory and counter-identificatory aspects, simultaneously creating a distance from other people, death and illness and a closeness to health, happiness and success. This kind of portrayal creates a binary opposition between a negative and a positive HIV status.

The material I have analysed indicates that the goal and ideal is to fully accept HIV and regard it as something that eventually enriches life and to become someone who is living a healthy and happy life. In the HIV narrative, the protagonists are shaped through identification and things that are given positive value. However, the protagonists are also shaped using counter-identifications and distancing from things that are regarded as negative. This shaping of the protagonists carves a hero narrative of, if not a physical, then a social and emotional hero.

Counter-identifications: not being sad, HIV not being a trauma

The medical bodily perspective of the life-and-death binary related to HIV is an important focus of *The Longest Journey Is the Journey Within – The Film about Steve*. The medications are described as miracles and the medical facilities in Stockholm that used to house the HIV ward have been transformed into a maternity ward, a transformation that Steve describes as "just amazing. The place is full of life now, and that feels nice."

In the middle of the film, Staffan Hildebrand asks Steve Sjöquist: "Is HIV/AIDS an important issue in Sweden today?" Steve states:

> It's a really important issue. We're a rich country, and we travel all around the world. Young people go to study on the other side of the world. We go to countries where HIV is very common, so we'll have to deal with for a long time, and it's important that we keep talking about it.

In the film different people engaged in the issue of HIV and AIDS are also being interviewed. The film is mainly portraying a historical exposé and the AIDS crisis in the 1980s and 1990s in Sweden or ongoing struggles and new cases of HIV worldwide. Steve is describing his partner, who took his own life: "He also lived with HIV, but he couldn't deal with life anymore". How HIV was a factor in that situation the film does not explain. In the film there is not much about everyday life with HIV or moments when HIV becomes evident. Portrayal of obstacles in encounters with other people or the health-care sector, physically or emotionally is not in focus. This picture and representation might give the viewer the impression that living with HIV in Sweden today is not a challenging experience, since there is HIV medication and free-of-charge health care. Even though grief is a strong theme in the film, especially when portraying the 1980s and 1990s, but also in relation to the recent loss of partner, the portrayal of HIV as a contemporary Swedish phenomenon has a strong positive and hopeful theme. And even though challenges of living with HIV is being touched upon, when Steve says that he is meeting people with HIV that do not dare to talk to other people about them having HIV, and that "we still have a lot left to do". Except for the interview with HIV activist Simon Blom, who is stating that he has physical effects with HIV, the representation of people with HIV having difficulties living with HIV are not included. The narrative, hence, is in line with normalisation strategies designed to give HIV and people with HIV more positive connotations. In focus are a survivor narrative and a success story of a strong hero. This way of portraying and representing HIV might exclude contemporary experiences of trauma, shame and fear that a life with HIV might still entail despite the medical developments (Ljungcrantz 2017). When portraying HIV as an illness to live with, which in a contemporary Swedish context is foremost associated with hope, positivity and learning outcomes, Hildebrand contributes to a positive representation of HIV. This might have the effect of changing the negative discourse around HIV, which contributes to creating the HIV stigma, reproducing shame and fear and silence around experiences of living with HIV. Nevertheless, a representation that distances itself from the contemporary negative aspects of HIV, as an experienced trauma, might risk creating a distance to the kinds of experiences that are not positive or affirmative. Consequently, HIV is complex, and representing it needs to be complex as well, performing a balancing act that works against an HIV stigma while not erasing the problems and vulnerabilities that do exist and are experienced by people with HIV. An altogether positive representation might thus hide society's problems (Ahmed 2004: 200–202), in this case with HIV.

In this vein of hope and positivity, I recall a passage from the end of *Mitt positiva liv*, in which Andreas concludes that there is always hope and that there is always somebody who has a worse situation in life than oneself. The privileged position with free-of-charge health care and effective HIV medication is argued as a reason not to experience HIV as a trauma, a perspective gained after travelling in Zambia:

Sure, it's okay to be depressed sometimes. Be depressed and feel down. But I don't like to complain, and it has never been interesting to me that others should feel sorry for me. Those people who see themselves as victims and make the illness or something that they have been suffering from into a life-style of whining – they should go to Zambia. Because no matter how ter-rible the existence might be, there is always someone in a worse situation. And no matter how dark it might seem, there is always a glimmer of hope somewhere for those who search for it.

(Lundstedt and Blankens 2012: 237)

This portrayal has the effect of not only distancing the protagonist from suffering but of condemning people who still experience HIV as a trauma or something that complicates life and perhaps makes us depressed (see Ljungcrantz 2017).

In one of the scenes concluding the film, Staffan Hildebrand asks Steve Sjöquist what the most important thing he has learned from his work with HIV and AIDS is. Steve declares:

That nothing that's human is dangerous to talk about. There are so many things that we don't communicate about. And we think that we're all alone. But if you embrace your humanity and communicate openly…. You don't have to vent all your personal stuff, but we should talk about all the things we share as humans. I've learned that it's a lot easier to share your grief and happiness. When I asked to be included, when I was ill, I got to be included.

The necessity for people in a society to talk about difficult issues is raised in the documentary. However, where the boundary lies between what to talk about and what to avoid is a bit uncertain. Which issues can be regarded as common to human beings and which are not, and what might be defined as too personal, are questions to be discussed in relation to this quote. In consciousness-raising pro-ductions and representations, it is important to scrutinise various kinds of inclu-sions and exclusions, good examples and discouraging examples, in order to be able to carve out how meaning-making processes are being produced.

Belonging: normative lines and social categorisation between normality and deviation

When analysing identifications, social categorisation is a part of the internal identification, i.e. how a person is identifying, with what and whom. External identification, how other people see you and categorise you, also connects to social categorisations (see e.g. Fuss 1995; Butler 1997; Muñoz 1999; Lykke 2010). When analysing representations of HIV, I searched for connections to social categorisations or identity markers. Some of these markers can be explicit, when someone is stating that they are x or y. Others might be implicit, and this is what I as a viewer interprets from "reading between the lines", as how some-thing or someone appears. Evidently, it would be possible to search for more information elsewhere, but I am focusing on the film. Steve's Christian religious view becomes apparent when he mentions his profession as a deacon. When the deviations in relation to normativities are not mentioned, a person is imagined to be placed within the frames of normality. Therefore, when Steve on the one hand is outspoken as being homosexual, on the other hand he is probably believed to be not a substance user and to be a cis-man. Cis means on the same side, and relates to a person following normative lines when it comes to sex and gender, i.e. a person whose biological sex, legal sex, gender identity and gender expression follow the same line, while not following these lines is the definition of trans. However, this interpretation by the viewer happens in relation to previous knowledge, the historical imaginaries of HIV in which HIV is linked with the categorisation of people with HIV as associated with gay men, substance users and sex workers (see e.g. Bredström 2008; Johannisson 2002; Nilsson Schönnesson 2001; Thorsén 2013). Steve might then be imagined as a gay man. When analysing HIV in a Swedish context, normativities of whiteness and Swedishness become relevant (Bredström 2008; Ljungcrantz 2017). Visually, Steve has a white skin and he sounds like a native Swedish speaker. However, HIV is imagined as being associated with "the Others", with people already regarded as deviant, not only transgressing the normative boundaries of middle-class identity and heteronormative respectability but also with Swedishness and whiteness (Ljungcrantz 2017). Whiteness and Swedishness can be seen as processes of exclusion and inclusion, creating different forms of privilege for the people passing visually and behaviourally as conforming to the normativity (see e.g. Ahmed 2006; Mattsson 2005; Hübinette and Lundström 2011).

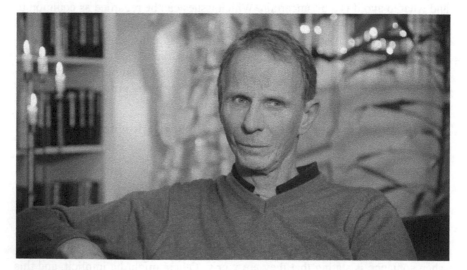

Figure 7.2 Steve Sjöquist. *The Longest Journey Is the Journey Within.*
Source: Hildebrand 2015.

In the cultural imaginaries, HIV has been constructed as a phenomenon that does not affect the general public but only a deviant minority. The portrayal of Steve also produces a closeness between HIV and certain lines of normality, which might open up the cultural imaginaries of HIV as being relevant to more people. However, at the same time as the reproduction of HIV is presented as acceptable for some people, who are following respectable normative lines, other aspects are deemed unacceptable: suffering, promiscuity, lack of education etc. Along these lines, belonging is an important word (Kafer 2013) and we might ask ourselves: To whom does HIV belong today? Where do people with HIV belong?

Conclusion

Normality and deviation are constructed in different ways in the documentary and the autobiographies; through linguistics, visuals and embodiment. An intersectional analysis shows the closeness and distance to different social categorisations. *The Longest Journey Is the Journey Within– The Film about Steve* is a story about the biographical aspect of a survivor. From the perspective of the film, it seems that HIV is still narrated with a strong focus on the disease aspect, instead of going more into the illness aspect and more experiential and everyday perspectives of having HIV. When documenting the historical context and medical developments around HIV, and hence the process of its transformation from a deadly into a chronic illness, there is a tendency to get stuck in the medical framework.

Normativities and deviations are negotiated in the film through portraits of distance and closeness, identificatory narratives and counter-identifications. Normativities and deviations are narrated in relation to and as being negotiated in line with wellness ideas, a strong neo-liberal subject and hero narratives that align with respectability and happiness. Read together with the autobiographies *Ophelias resa* and *Mitt positiva liv*, contemporary HIV narratives emerge as normalising HIV and potentially transforming it. HIV narratives that portray a survivor and a hero also tend to function as border-making narratives that risk excluding people who are not regarded or labelled as respectable. There is a transition from a positive touch and a strong personality into a narrative that performs wellness, both orienting towards creating the HIV-positive person as nowadays healthy and happy, and creating a division back in time between strong, positive survivors and weak, dying individuals.

The complexities of representing people with HIV becomes clear when analysing these biographical accounts, especially the portrayal of Steve in *The Longest Journey Is the Journey Within – The Film about Steve*. This is but a small part of the Face of AIDS film archive and the significance of the archive is the documentation of many faces of AIDS and HIV. However, in a Swedish context, where few people are open in public about their HIV diagnosis, the few who are almost inevitably become "the only face of HIV". With that said, I am longing for more faces to be seen, and that society might shift its prejudices against HIV and against people categorised as "the Other". This calls for critical reflections of the reproduction of "us" and "them" and how normativities are in play creating a distance between certain ways of living and being that HIV might enhance. The cultural imaginary of the normative majority vis-à-vis the deviant minority needs to be dealt with to enable more inclusive and nuanced stories of HIV. Nuanced stories about HIV and having HIV can be crucial, not only for changing the cultural imaginaries but also for influencing the lives of people with HIV, including many ways of living with the disease: more voices and perspectives are needed, including the suffering dimensions of a life with HIV, and different belongings in relation to social categorisations.

Representations and portrayals of people with HIV are important since they both reflect and influence the cultural imaginaries of HIV. The flexibility and tolerance towards HIV in the cultural imaginaries seem to depend on who has or is imagined as having HIV (Ljungcrantz 2017). It is also evident that the general public does not regard HIV as non-dramatic and the stigma containing fear and shame still seems to exist (Lindberg *et al.* 2015; Ljungcrantz 2017). This also pinpoints the idea of the task for a person representing HIV, becoming an HIV ambassador and the balancing act between widen the general public's ideas of HIV and including nuances of how it might be to live with HIV. We could be inspired by this analysis. However, the responsibility should rather be a task of the one's portraying HIV, for example government agencies working with HIV, than individuals having HIV. Once again, the complexities in representing HIV become clear; that is, how to create representations that enable people living with HIV to be regarded as both ordinary people and people who are in different ways affected by HIV. It is crucial to do both in order to open up the possibility of reacting to cultural imaginaries and discourses on HIV without subscribing to them, which risks shutting the doors on people and experiences that also belong here.

Note

1 The film can be regarded as part of a consciousness-raising and activist practice of which the filmmaker, Staffan Hildebrand, and the main character, Steve Sjöquist, have been, and still are, a part. For this I would like to thank them.

References

Ahmed, Sara (2004). *The Cultural Politics of Emotion*. Edinburgh: Edinburgh University Press.
Ahmed, Sara (2006). *Queer Phenomenology: Orientations, Objects, Others*. New York and London: Routledge.
Berlant, Lauren and Warner, Michael (1998). "Sex in Public", *Critical Inquiry*, 24(2): 547–566.
Bredström, Anna (2008). *Safe Sex, Unsafe Identities: Intersections of "Race", Gender and Sexuality in Swedish HIV/AIDS Policy*. Dissertation. Linköping: Linköping University Press.
Bremer, Signe (2011). *Kroppslinjer. Kön, transsexualism och kropp i berättelser om könskorrigering*. Dissertation. Göteborg and Stockholm: Makadam förlag.

Butler, Judith (1990). *Gender Trouble: Feminism and the Subversion of Identity*. New York and London: Taylor & Francis.

Butler, Judith (1997). *Excitable Speech: A Politics of the Performative*. New York: Routledge.

Cederström, Carl and André Spicer (2015). *The Wellness Syndrome*. Cambridge: Polity.

Connell, Raewyn (2010). "Understanding Neoliberalism", in Susan Braedley and Meg Luxton (eds), *Neoliberalism and Everyday Life*. Montreal: McGill-Queen's University Press.

Couser, G. Thomas (1997). *Recovering Bodies: Illness, Disability, and Life Writing*. Madison, WI: University of Wisconsin Press.

Couser, G. Thomas (2010). *Corporealities: Discourses of Disability, Signifying Bodies, Disability in Contemporary Life Writing*. Ann Arbor, MI: University of Michigan Press.

Dawson, Graham (1994). *Soldier Heroes. British Adventure, Empire and the Imagining of Masculinity*. London: Routledge.

Edelman, Lee (2004). *No Future: Queer Theory and Death Drive*. Durham, NC, and London: Duke University Press.

Ehrenreich, Barbara (2009). *Smile or Die: How Positive Thinking Fooled America and the World*. London: Granta.

Eriksson, Lars E. (2012). *Positivt liv. En internationell kunskapsöversikt om att undersöka livskvalitet och livssituation hos personer som lever med hiv*. Solna: Smittskyddsinstitutet.

Frank, Arthur W. (1995). *The Wounded Storyteller: Body, Illness, and Ethics*. Chicago, IL: University of Chicago Press.

Fuss, Diana (1995). *Identification Papers*. New York: Routledge.

Gustavson, Malena (2006). *Blandade känslor. Bisexuella kvinnors praktik och politik*. Dissertation. Göteborg: Kabusa.

Halberstam, J. Jack (2005). *In a Queer Time and Place: Transgender Bodies, Subcultural Lives*. London: New York Press.

Hübinette, Tobias and Catrin Lundström (2011). "Sweden after the Recent Election: The Double-Binding Power of Swedish Whiteness through the Mourning of the Loss of 'Old Sweden' and the Passing of 'Good Sweden'", *NORA – Nordic Journal of Feminist and Gender Research*, 19(1): 42–52.

Johannisson, Karin (2002). *Medicinens öga. Sjukdom, medicin och samhälle – historiska erfarenheter*. 2nd ed. Stockholm: Norstedts.

Jurecic, Ann (2012). *Illness as Narrative*. Pittsburgh, PA: University of Pittsburgh Press.

Kafer, Alison (2013). *Feminist, Queer, Crip*. Bloomington, IN: Indiana University Press.

Kean, Jessica (2015). "A Stunning Plurality: Unravelling Hetero- and Mononormativities through HBO's Big Love", *Sexualities*, 18(5–6): 698–713.

Kleinman, Arthur (1988). *The Illness Narratives: Suffering, Healing, and the Human Condition*. New York: Basic.

Larsson, Agneta and Ophelia Haanyama Ørum (2007). *Ophelias resa*. Stockholm: Bokförlaget Atlas.

Lindberg, Maria, Lena Wettergren, Maria Wiklander, Veronica Svedhem-Johansson and Lars E. Eriksson (2014). "Psychometric Evaluation of the HIV Stigma Scale in a Swedish Context", *PLoS ONE*, 9(12): 1–16.

Ljungcrantz, Desireé (2017). *Skrubbsår. Berättelser om föreställningar och erfarenheter av hiv i samtida Sverige*. Göteborg: Makadam förlag.

Lundstedt, Andreas and Cecilia Blankens (2012). *Mitt positiva liv*. Stockholm: Norstedts.

118   *Desireé Ljungcrantz*

Lupton, Deborah (2003). *Medicine as Culture: Illness, Disease and the Body in Western Societies*. 2nd ed. London: Sage.

Luxton, Meg (2010). "Doing Neoliberalism: Perverse Individualism in Personal Life", in Susan Braedley and Meg Luxton (eds), *Neoliberalism and Everyday Life*. Montreal: McGill-Queen's University Press.

Lykke, Nina (2010). *Feminist Studies: A Guide to Intersectional Theory, Methodology and Writing*. London: Routledge.

Mattsson, Katarina (2005). "Diskrimineringens andra ansikte. Svenskhet och 'det vita väster ländska'", in Paulina de los Reyes and Masoud Kamali (eds), *Bortom Vi och Dom. Teoretiska reflektioner om makt, integration och strukturell diskriminering*. SOU 2005:41.

McRuer, Robert (2006). "Compulsory Able-Bodiedness and Queer/Disabled Existence", in Lennard J. Davis (ed.), *The Disability Studies Reader*. 2nd ed. London and New York: Routledge.

Muñoz, José Esteban (1999). *Disidentifications: Queers of Color and the Performance of Politics*. Minneapolis, MN: University of Minnesota Press.

Nilsson Schönnesson, Lena (2001). *Med livet i fokus. Strategier hos kvinnor och män med hiv för att återerövra livskvalitet*. Solna: Folkhälsoinstitutet.

Patton, Cindy (1990). *Inventing AIDS*. New York: Routledge.

Roseneil, Sasha (2006). "On Not Living with a Partner: Unpicking Coupledom and Cohabitation", *Sociological Research Online*, 11(3): 1–14.

Rubin, Gayle (1984). "Thinking Sex: Notes towards a Radical Theory of the Politics of Sexuality", in Carole S. Vance (ed.), *Pleasure and Danger: Exploring Female Sexuality*. Boston, MA: Routledge & Kegan Paul.

Rydström, Jens (2008). "Legalizing Love in a Cold Climate: The History, Consequences and Recent Developments of Registered Partnerships in Scandinavia", *Sexualities*, 11(1–2): 193–226.

Rydström, Lise-Lotte (2015). *Health-Related Quality of Life and HIV-Related Stigma in Children Living with HIV in Sweden*. Dissertation. Stockholm: Karolinska Institutet.

Skeggs, Beverly (1997). *Formations of Class and Gender: Becoming Respectable*. London: Sage.

Svenaeus, Fredrik (2013). *Homo patologicus. Medicinska diagnoser i vår tid*. Hägersten: Tankekraft.

Svensson, Ingeborg (2013). *Liket i garderoben. Bögar, begravningar och 80-talets hivepidemi*. New ed. Dissertation. Stockholm: Ordfront/Normal förlag.

SFS 2004:168. Sveriges riksdag. *Smittskyddslag* [Contagious Disease Act].

SFS 162:700. Sveriges riksdag. *Brottsbalken* [Penal Code].

The Ethical Council, Linköping (2016). www.epn.se/linkoeping/om-naemnden, last accessed 30 January 2017.

The Public Health Agency of Sweden (2013). *Bakgrundstexter presenterade vid SMI:s och RAV:s workshop den 11 september 2012*, www.sls.se/Global/RAV/Dokument/bakgrundstexter-smittsamhet-vid-behandlad-hivinfektion.pdf, last accessed 30 January 2017.

The Public Health Agency of Sweden (2016). *Information and Statistics*, www.folkhal somyndigheten.se/folkhalsorapportering-statistik/statistikdatabaseroch-visualisering/sjukdomsstatistik/hivinfektion, last accessed 30 January 2017.

The Public Health Agency of Sweden and the National Board of Health and Welfare (2010). *Hiv, STI och juridik i Sverige*, www.folkhalsomyndigheten.se/pagefiles/12837/hiv-stijuridik- sverige-176–2010.pdf, last accessed 5 February 2015 (no longer accessible).

Thorsén, David (2013). *Den svenska aidsepidemin. Ankomst, bemötande, innebörd.* Dissertation. Uppsala: Uppsala University.
Treichler, Paula A. (1999). *How to Have Theory in an Epidemic: Cultural Chronicles of AIDS*, Durham, NC: Duke University Press.
UNAIDS (2015). *AIDS by the Numbers 2015*, www.unaids.org/sites/default/files/media_asset/AIDS_by_the_numbers_2015_en.pdf, last accessed 25 November 2017.
UNAIDS (2016). *Fact Sheet November 2016*, www.unaids.org/en/ resources/fact-sheet, last accessed 30 January 2017.
Weait, Matthew (2011). "The Criminalisation of HIV Exposure and Transmission: A Global Review", *Working Paper Prepared for the Third Meeting of the Technical Advisory Group*. Global Commission on HIV and the Law, 7–9 July 2011, http://hiv lawcommission.org/index.php/report-working-papers?task=document.viewdoc&id=90, last accessed 30 January 2017.

Films

Hildebrand, Staffan, *The Longest Journey Is the Journey Within – The Film about Steve* (2015).

Part III
Stigma and trauma

8 Waiting for a cure

Cultural perspectives on AIDS in the 1980s

Adam Brenthel and Kristofer Hansson

We begin this chapter with a return to 1988 and a Parisian hospital with a patient room with no patient. Instead, a doctor, Didier Jayle, is there, interviewed by the Swedish film director and journalist Staffan Hildebrand. The interview is conducted in the room and the doctor is sitting on the bed, the same bed where a patient died only three hours earlier, according to the doctor. He seems to be relaxed and under his white coat he wears a shirt and tie. It is still early in the history of AIDS and doctors and their patients are waiting for a cure. Hildebrand seems somewhat puzzled about this and asks the doctor: "In this room, your patient died, how do you prepare the patients for dying?" The doctor hesitates for a second and, instead of letting him answer, Hildebrand asks again, now more intensely: "When you know the patients will die soon, how do you prepare them?" It is the peak of the AIDS epidemic in Paris and there is not much more the doctors can do apart from preparing the young patients to die. Jayle answers:

> AIDS is a war. And we are fighting with the patients against the virus. And it is horrible to see young people dying from AIDS. And here in this room there was a young guy, thirty-two years old, who died. And it is impossible to carry on, to carry on like that. And we have to tell, to alarm, young people to be very cautious in their lives, not to die of AIDS.
>
> (Archive ID: 1988_102)[1]

In this short sequence – four minutes and thirty-nine seconds of unedited film – the camera focuses on the doctor. This male doctor is doing most of the talking; his gaze is directed into the camera. Hildebrand has thus created a medical environment that we can recognize culturally. There is the male doctor, with a white coat, in a patient room that has a bed. The doctor is furthermore expected to have the answers to the questions that are asked. At the same time, there is one thing in this setting that makes us all uneasy, and it apparently also makes the doctor uneasy. This is a patient room that is empty of patients. At this time, in 1988, there is no cure and young people die and leave rooms empty.

The aim of this chapter is to study *waiting as a cultural practice* in the medical context at the end of the 1980s. It might, for example, be a case of waiting for a young person to die while waiting for a cure. It might also concern expectations on how you should be waiting. Hildebrand's intense question to the doctor is not only about how the patient is prepared for dying; the question itself also reveals that the waiting is complicated. How is waiting framed in Hildebrand's filming? How is it visually expressed and how do Hildebrand and the persons he talks to incarnate it in speech and bodily expressions? These questions are dealt with in this chapter with the help of a number of recordings from the Face of AIDS film archive.

The Face of AIDS film archive

The chapter presents and analyses a number of unedited documentary sequences that Hildebrand shot in 1988. Together with cameraman Christer Strandell, he traveled around the world to make the opening film for the Fourth International AIDS Conference, in Stockholm in June 1988. The result, *Crossover: The Global Impact of AIDS*, was shown at the conference, but as Hildebrand points out this was also the start of the Face of AIDS film archive. Hildebrand was given the assignment by Dr. Hans Wigzell at Karolinska Institutet, not only to make the opening film but also to document the impact of AIDS on a global scale. Hildebrand therefore returned to the subject over and over again, producing many hours of film. Hildebrand writes about Wigzell's wish that "[h]e wanted to develop a film archive on this new human epidemic, and he wanted me to do the job."[2]

For this reason, much of the material in the archive is unedited. We find interviews that end in the middle of a sentence, poor sound, retakes, a cameraman testing different camera angles and so on. The archive could easily lend itself to claims of truth in line with a traditional documentary genre, and it presents itself as close to a "truth." We have, however, analyzed the films as expressions of a reality that Hildebrand, Strandell and the individuals that they film are constructing together in a specific historical context. This is a time when the promises of the golden age of medicine were challenged and plague was once again a chilling word. It is, with other words, the specific situation that has constructed the specific archive artefact (Frykman and Gilje 2003). At the same time, there is a delayed transmission of the past – of the situation in 1988 – when we now analyze the sequences of the films in this chapter (Ernst 2015) – and still we see similarities with our present time.

There are, at the time for our analysis (the spring of 2017), 221 film sequences in the archive from the year 1988. It was never our ambition to present and analyze all sequences. Instead we are interested in making a small incision in the material to understand how waiting is negotiated and performed by the doctors who were left with no alternative. Our material has thus been limited by the selection "Attitude of Health Personnel" in the Medical Subject Headings (MeSH) of the archive. This selection resulted in six film sequences, which were filmed in the U.S.A., France, Italy and Australia. Two of these were eliminated because they were not available to us via the online archive platform. The remaining ones are two films featuring Dr. Didier Jayle from France, one film featuring Dr. Paul Volberding from the U.S.A. and one dialogue between Lyle Taylor, who in 1988 was dying of AIDS, and his doctor, John Dwyer, at the Prince of Wales Hospital in Sydney. This provided film material of a total duration of fifty minutes and thirty-two seconds. We have viewed this material several times to analyze what they talk about and how Hildebrand and Strandell visualize the conversations.

To conceptualize an emerging disease

When AIDS appeared in the 1980s, it challenged our perceptions of what medicine actually could do. There had been other events that strongly questioned the hope that society had put into medicine, for instance the thalidomide scandal in the 1960s. What was special about AIDS was that the virus potentially could affect everybody and medicine seemed to have no remedy to offer. The very first known cases were detected in 1981 and only two years later nearly 3,000 people had died, a number that would increase exponentially in the coming years. This affected many young people as Dr. Didier Jayle expressed in the scene quoted above. The fact that young people died made this an even larger failure for medicine. Dr. Paul Volberding from the U.S.A. reflects upon this when he says:

> I think one of the things that we hopefully have learned is that, we came into this with a certain incredible ignorance. There was the feeling that we could solve any problem. That basically, we had solved all problems of infections. And yet something like this comes and teaches us, how ignorant we were and how humble we should be for the future.
>
> (Archive ID: 1988_194)

The resurgence of the research field concerning emerging or re-emerging infectious diseases can be seen as an answer to this development where AIDS is only one example (Washer 2010). From the 1980s and onwards, infectious diseases have become a new medical, cultural and social phenomenon, and the discourses of this phenomenon can be found in for example popular culture. There have been many infectious diseases identified since the beginning of the 1970s that have made something of a cultural impact. Besides AIDS, there have been Ebola, hepatitis C and SARS, to mention a few (Satcher 1995). Medicine does not have a cure for every virus or bacteria anymore, instead there is a growing pessimism in reference to what medicine can do in the long run. These medical challenges are addressed within medical research today, but it is also becoming a central theme for medical humanities as the emerging infectious diseases we face today also change how we culturally and socially, but also bodily, relate to health and death. The growing pessimism is therefore significant for cultural expectations of what we think medicine can or cannot do. Many of the emerging or re-emerging infectious diseases are represented through news media. Peter Washer, a researcher in the philosophy of science, claims that this is how lay-people learn more about the diseases (Washer 2004). A central topic in this conceptualization has been a form of "Othering," where the Western audience creates a distance to the threat posed by for example AIDS, Ebola or SARS. In relation to AIDS, Washer writes that another function of the new disease is to:

> apportion blame by constructing boundaries between self and "other," with misfortunes understood to be the price paid by people who are bad, dirty, bizarre, promiscuous; people who are "not like us." AIDS, for example, was initially configured in terms of earlier epidemics which had been linked to foreigners, out groups and perverse practices.
>
> (Washer 2005: 3)

But this idea also provides what Washer calls a collective coping mechanism that helps people to categorize new diseases and the danger they might bring to the individual and to the society at large (Washer 2005). Mass media is one way to study the development of diseases and how society copes with them, often with a risk perspective (Beck 1992). In this chapter, we want to present a different theoretical perspective that focuses more on existential questions that come with emerging or re-emerging infectious diseases. The reason for this is that there are other questions that are not about "othering" or risk, for example regarding how to deal with death. Questions about death also concern being cured and whether medical research might find a way to stop the emerging diseases, both for the infected individual and for the society at risk. A central question connected to this is how to negotiate the situation of waiting to die – when there is nothing more anybody can do.

Waiting for death

How do we handle waiting in a culture that always tries to have a solution to everything? Ethnologists Orvar Löfgren and Billy Ehn pose the question of "what kind of 'doing nothing' constitutes waiting" (Löfgren and Ehn 2010: 10)? One way to deal with it is to camouflage the waiting with other not-so-meaningful tasks. If we are sitting in the doctor's waiting room, we might be reading meaningless magazines to "kill time." While waiting for the bus, we will pick up our mobile phones to see once again that no one is trying to get in touch with us. But what happens when we wait for death? When there is no cure for the disease and all that remains is to wait for the body to give up – when the disease puts life in brackets? To do absolutely nothing, except to wait for death, is challenging in a culture like ours that values achievement, meaning and development. You would want to achieve good health or you will be helped to die with dignity (Alftberg and Hansson 2012). If we go back to the interview with Didier Jayle, we can see how waiting for a patient's death is expressed through what is said and how it is filmed.

Strandell's film sequence, in which Hildebrand asks his question about how the patients are prepared, starts by showing a small bedside table. It is a scene that is less than five seconds long, after which the camera pans over to the

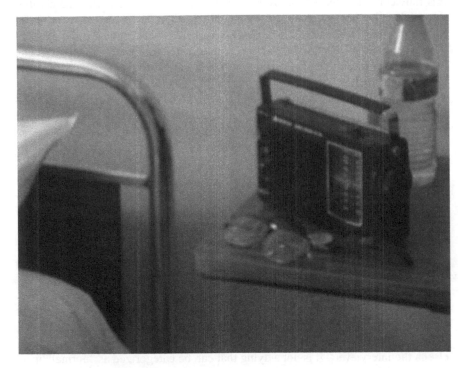

Figure 8.1 Fragments of a life.
Source: Archive ID 1988_102.

doctor. The film almost stops during these five seconds and the moving picture resembles a still life. On the table, there is a plastic bottle with almost all the water left, there is a radio and, in front of this, there are a pair of glasses and a wristwatch. These things are not simply passive objects in a still life, but instead objects used by Hildebrand and Strandell to give the documentary a direction (Miller 2010). Through this still life we can raise questions about the purpose of this picture for Hildebrand and Strandell. What can the still life tell us?

From a purely aesthetic point of view, one might answer that Hildebrand and Strandell are using the objects to capture the impatience of what is happening in Paris and in the world. They use them as fragments of a lived life to frame the question of how the doctors are preparing the young people for death. The watch can here be seen as a symbol for time that can never be stopped. Even if another young patient is now dead, time still continues inexorably, along with the waiting for a cure.

This almost still sequence can be seen as a social representation of how Hildebrand and Strandell want to visually frame the question of how the doctors prepare the young people that are soon to die. Through values, ideas and metaphors in this film sequence and the interview, different social representations at this time come to life. We can follow Peter Washer's method when he clarifies that "[s]ocial representations are best studied when 'new' concerns arise for different groups" (Washer 2005: 2). AIDS was this "new" concern; the dying of young people was something that was a failure for medicine. All these young people who died and the few belongings they seemed to leave behind in empty hospital rooms.

In the next sequence, the doctor is back on screen again and answers Hildebrand's question. This sequence begins with the camera zooming in on the doctor until he becomes a talking head. The doctor says:

> You know, doctors are not very well prepared to speak of death and especially in dermatology. We are not accustomed to see people dying when they come to the hospital and we have to ask new questions, to change our practice to be able to help patients to fight, and if we don't succeed and they die in hospital sometimes, or they die at home and we have to be there with the patient to the last minute, that's what we have to do.
>
> (Archive ID: 1988_102)

Death is a central theme in many of Hildebrand's interviews in the 1980s. When talking about it, the doctors always arrive at the impossibility of actually handling it when there is no cure. They are not used to seeing young people die, at least not without the possibility to do something. Death becomes something else in the interviews – it is not a dying that can be categorized as "normal" in an era of modern medicine. At this time, it was not known if the disease would escalate or stop. Jayle's pessimism is therefore also about not knowing or being able to predict the future, not knowing if a remedy would come. This resulted in a form of waiting that seems to leave the doctor with a feeling of frustration; he wants to do so much but he does not have the tools, except his presence, to be "with the patient to the last minute."

This sense of frustration and the situation of waiting should not be seen as something that Jayle constructed himself; it is also a representation constructed together with Hildebrand's question and the filming. "[H]ow do you prepare them?" Hildebrand asks, a question that could also be understood as a question about how to wait for death.

The conversation between Lyle Taylor and his doctor, John Dwyer, at the Prince of Wales Hospital in Sydney addresses a similar theme. Six minutes and thirty seconds into the sequence, Hildebrand asks the question "Do you regard the threat now as a dangerous problem to the world?" – and it is not the actual answer but the way the doctor answers that is telling. The camera frames Dwyer in a medium shot. He is dressed as the typical doctor in a white coat and in the background, we see an empty hospital bed. We also see Taylor's leg in the scene as Dwyer begins to answer, giving the sequence an out-of-the-ordinary feeling.

> AIDS is the black plague of our time, no question about that, it devastates the immune system and with that immune system destroyed, all these

consequences are visited upon people. It is a most serious epidemic. Unless we control it, it will take thousands of more lives in the next few years, already we have lost more than two million years of productive young life to this virus. And we feel privileged to deal with the lives of this world, but you can imagine the frustration we have, because, as he knows, there is very little we can do for him at this moment, unfortunately.

(Archive ID: 1988_25)

It is strange, and we feel uncomfortable to watch a sequence where the doctor is saying to the camera that he cannot do enough for the patient, or maybe nothing, with the very same patient present in the room. Normally the doctor should say that they would do everything to help the young man. That is at least what we expect culturally. However, "at this moment" in history, as the doctor says, they can only wait, wait for a better treatment or wait for the patient to die. This is frustrating for Dwyer because he sees all the lives going to waste in this epidemic. The interview is made more poignant by the fact, stated in the meta-data accompanying the film, that the patient Lyle Taylor died ten hours after the interview.

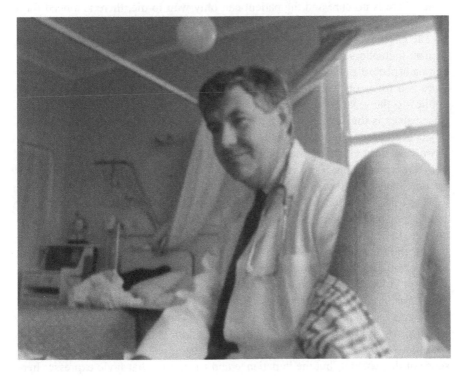

Figure 8.2 The patient present in the same room.
Source: Archive ID 1988_25.

Metaphors of time

A social representation that becomes central in the interview above is the way the virus is described in terms of war. Metaphors are a common social representation of diseases, and extensive research has been conducted in the field (Gustafsson and Hommerberg 2016). Susan Sontag was one of the earliest writers to discuss how diseases like cancer and AIDS are understood, based on metaphors of war (Sontag 1990). Rather often this war is expressed in popular culture, and it is a war that can be fought both by those who are affected by the disease and by professional medicine. The metaphors used are clear and often directly linked to the virus as an enemy. The body of the patient then becomes a veritable battlefield and the metaphor points out either winners or losers in a race against time.

For emerging or re-emerging infectious diseases, metaphors are used as a way of anchoring what is said about the diseases. In this way, the metaphors enable the listener to understand; a relation is created to what is already known and understood (Washer 2005). AIDS then becomes one of those diseases that has similarities with other diseases that are described as a battle or war. The patients become types in an almost "archetypal myth" for our society (Hawkins 1999). But, instead of seeing them as myths, we argue here that the metaphors are a cultural response to a situation in which there is little hope for the persons involved. When there is no cure and the patient can only wait to die, there is a need for a language to handle this, to say the least, existential crisis.

The cognitive linguists and philosophers George Lakoff and Mark Johnson explain metaphors as meanings and associations from one domain that create a certain aspect of reality in another (Lakoff and Johnson 1980). In their analysis, there is a focus on words and sentences. However, their argument can also be applied to the creation of reality through filming; one example given earlier in this chapter is the sequence with the wristwatch. Accordingly, the watch as an object becomes a symbol that gives the viewer a certain notion of time as central if we want to understand the reality of AIDS. In this way, the watch becomes both a representation of the young man who recently died, but also a symbol for the time that is lost through all the young deaths.

It is this dimension of time that becomes central for understanding Didier Jayle's perspective that "AIDS is a war," mentioned in the beginning of this chapter. In one way, he is anchoring AIDS as an emerging disease – a virus – that he and the patient are at war with, and which needs to be fought. It is also a fight because the people who die are young and had a future, but AIDS entails a situation in which time seems to run out for them. The metaphor thus reinforces the distrust that Jayle seems to feel to this new situation when he says: "And it is horrible to see young people dying from AIDS. And here in this room there was a young guy, thirty-two years old, who died. And it is impossible to carry on, *to carry on like that*" (Archive ID:1988_102, our emphasis). It goes beyond the scope of this chapter, but the impatience and frustration that Jayle expresses here were also an important part of the AIDS activism that arose in the 1980s (Treichler 1999).

Metaphors for AIDS were thus not only constructed by Jayle and the other doctors; Hildebrand and Strandell were also instrumental by posing questions and placing the camera. In the interview with Paul Volberding, this becomes even more obvious. In the sequence, we see Volberding – filmed in a medium shot – in shirt and tie. He is a little bit older than Jayle but could still be categorized as a young doctor in the middle of his life. Volberding is sitting in his office and in the background we see his many diplomas. Almost ten minutes into the interview, Hildebrand asks the question: "How does it feel for you as a doctor, not to be able to cure young, powerful, healthy patients and who start to develop AIDS"? We can see that this question is similar to the discussion with Jayle; it focuses on time, and young people are dying from AIDS. What is new in this question is the straightforwardness in Volberding's answer, maybe because he is a little bit more experienced than Jayle:

> My background is in cancer medicine, and I have a certain amount of training and expectations that my patients will die, cancer patients tend to die. What's different about AIDS is the youth of the patients. All of the patients, instead of being seventy or eighty years old, are twenty, thirty or forty years old, the same age that I am. That has an important set of problems, because usually I think that a physician can distance himself from the patient, sometimes continually, sometimes uncontinually, telling ourself "It's not me dying in this bed," of AIDS, once you come over the minor differences between someone's lifestyle and your own, you realise it could be you dying in the bed.
>
> (Archive ID: 1988_194)

Volberding answers more carefully, using other metaphors than Jayle; maybe this is consciously done. But what both doctors do, with the help of Hildebrand, is to construct a metaphor about time. Usually, time is somewhat abstract and we most often use metaphors to talk about time; we say that we spend time or we waste time as if time were money (Lakoff and Johnson 1980). In a similar way, seemingly, the dying young patients in the hospital beds become metaphors for the frailty of life. To understand this episode in 1988, Hildebrand is using a strong metaphor; to a large extent, this is about understanding that time is passing by in vain, while we are waiting for a cure.

But not only is time passing by for the individual lives; this metaphor is also connected to a narrative of morality when fighting AIDS. It is not only that time is passing by in a boring waiting process. Instead, time could here be seen as something that the medical staff should take responsibility for, by making life acceptable for the young people with AIDS. The doctors appearing in the sequences express that this could be too much of a burden for them to carry.

Conclusion: to take care of time

Waiting becomes central in the interviews and something that the doctors are reflecting upon in relation to the questions asked by Hildebrand. In 1988, people are waiting for any new treatment that will give the life back to young people that have AIDS. People are also fearing that this emerging infectious disease could spread and escalate. But, above all, people are waiting for death, all the young men in cities like Paris, New York and Stockholm, who are carrying the disease that will soon take their lives, and the burden is reflected by the doctors in the sequences. As it seems, the doctors identify with their patients, but they are supposed to carry on even after the death of their patients. Is it too much for them? Maybe. The Swedish author and comedian Jonas Gardell made this struggle palpable in his novel about two young men who find each other's love in Stockholm in the 1980s (Gardell 2012).[3] We follow them as they leave collective and societal expectations behind to create a new life outside of the closet. The waiting is over. But, instead of a free life, one of them contracts HIV and the story instead becomes a story of waiting for suffering and death. This is also described in ethnologist Ingeborg Svensson's study about gay men's funerals in the 1980s (Svensson 2007). The feeling of waiting that Gardell and Svensson capture, can also be used in our hermeneutic understanding of the waiting that is constructed in the documentary interviews.

We began this chapter with a quote by Jayle, where he pointed out, as a response to the question of how he tried to handle his waiting, that young people need to be cautious in their lives: "And we have to tell, to alarm, young people to be very cautious in their lives, not to die of AIDS" (Archive ID: 1988_102). The death of young men influenced Jayle and left him with a feeling that is also recurrently expressed in the books by Gardell and Svensson. This existential dimension is negotiated in the other interviews that have been analyzed in this chapter. In a shot where only Dr. Dwyer is seen in the frame, he talks about all the young people dying of AIDS, at that moment in 1988, as well as the patient Lyle Taylor, who is lying in bed just next to the doctor. Answering one of Hildebrand's questions, Dwyer talks about the lives that are lost because of the virus, and, as previously quoted, he continues to speak about the frustration he feels about the young lives that are now wasted.

> We feel privilege to deal with the life of this world, but you can imagine the frustration we have, because, as he knows, there is very little we can do for him at the moment unfortunately. Except enjoy his friendship and hopefully his respect, which we return manifold.
>
> (Archive ID: 1988_25)

Waiting for death, and the warlike metaphors that were used, forces us to believe that the young men's waiting was primarily seen as problematic. Waiting is many times pictured as something that reproduces a lot of different emotional aspects in relation to time that is moving slowly forward. As in our understanding of war, waiting becomes central and raises questions like when the bombing will start and why the enemies are not coming. However, there are also emotions that may be related to specific places. The different rooms in the hospital are such places where the experience of waiting becomes clear (Bournes and Mitchell 2002). Dwyer, Jayle and Volberding also experienced the meaning of waiting and the interviews express a profound care for the young people dying. In this way, there is a discourse in 1988 that is not only about AIDS as a new emerging disease but also a discourse on how to handle time.

In this chapter, we therefore conclude that waiting is a significant issue in understanding the cultural existential dimensions of emerging diseases. The way we handle the many dimensions of waiting is essential for how well we take care of the patients who are lying in their beds, facing death.

Notes

1 The transcribed material in our chapter has in some cases been grammar corrected in order to avoid misunderstandings when reading the text out of the context of its film.
2 Interview with Staffan Hildebrand in May 2015, Background material, Face of AIDS Film Archive, https://faceofaids.ki.se/archive/1988-crossover-short, last accessed September 24, 2017.
3 Is also to be seen in the miniseries *Don't Ever Wipe Tears without Gloves* (2012), directed by Simon Kaijser.

References

Alftberg, Åsa and Kristofer Hansson (2012). "Introduction: Self-Care Translated into Practice," *Culture Unbound*, 4: 415–424.
Beck, Ulrich (1992). *Risk Society: Towards a New Modernity*. London: Sage.
Bournes, Debra A. and Gail J. Mitchell (2002). "Waiting: The Experience of Persons in a Critical Care Waiting Room," *Research in Nursing & Health*, 25(1): 58–67.
Ernst, Wolfgang (2015). *Stirrings in the Archives: Order from Disorder*. Lanham, MD: Rowman & Littlefield.
Frykman, Jonas and Nils Gilje, eds. (2003). *Being There: New Perspectives on Phenomenology and the Analysis of Culture*. Lund: Nordic Academic Press.
Gardell, Jonas (2012). *Torka aldrig tårar utan handskar. 1, Kärleken*. Stockholm: Norstedt.
Gustafsson, Anna W. and Charlotte Hommerberg (2016). "'Pojken lyfter sitt svärd. Ger sig in i en strid han inte kan vinna': om metaforer och kronisk cancersjukdom," *Socialmedicinsk tidskrift*, 93(3): 271–270.
Hawkins, Anne Hunsaker (1999). *Reconstructing Illness: Studies in Pathography*. 2nd ed. West Lafayette, IN: Purdue University Press.
Lakoff, George and Mark Johnson (1980). *Metaphors We Live By*. Chicago, IL: University of Chicago Press.
Löfgren, Orvar and Billy Ehn (2010). *The Secret World of Doing Nothing*. Berkeley, CA: University of California Press.
Miller, Daniel (2010). *Stuff*. Cambridge: Polity Press.
Satcher, David (1995). "Emerging Infections: Getting Ahead of the Curve," *Emerging Infectious Diseases*, 1(1): 1–6.
Sontag, Susan (1990). *Illness as Metaphor; and, AIDS and Its Metaphors*. New York: Picador/Farrar, Straus and Giroux.
Svensson, Ingeborg (2007). *Liket i garderoben: en studie av sexualitet, livsstil och begravning*. Dissertation. Stockholm: Stockholms Universitet.

Treichler, Paula A. (1999). *How to Have Theory in an Epidemic: Cultural Chronicles of AIDS*. Durham, NC: Duke University Press.

Washer, Peter (2004). "Representations of SARS in the UK Newspapers," *Social Science and Medicine*, 59(12): 2561–2571.

Washer, Peter (2005). "Representations of 'Newly Emerging' Infectious Diseases in the British Newspapers," Unpublished paper, www.inter-disciplinary.net/ptb/mso/hid/hid4/Peter%20Washer%20-%20Oxford%20paper.pdf.

Washer, Peter (2010). *Emerging Infectious Diseases and Society*. Basingstoke: Palgrave Macmillan.

9 Social suffering as structural and symbolic violence

LGBT experiences in the Face of AIDS film archive[1]

Marco Bacio and Cirus Rinaldi

Introduction: structural and symbolic violence and LGBT issues – a transnational phenomenon

The cultural and sociological analysis of AIDS gives researchers the chance to consider the alarming concentration of HIV among vulnerable populations. Even if explicit discrimination has decreased at least in some Western countries, both in developed states – within their ethnic and racial minority groups and marginal populations (i.e., sex workers) – and in developing countries there are individuals living with HIV who experience structural and symbolic violence due to poverty, racism, sexism, homophobia/transphobia, gender inequality, social exclusion, stigmatization, or religious and sexual oppression (Farmer 2001; Parker 2002; Bourdieu 1990; 2001). This is especially true if we consider that the HIV/AIDS epidemic requires us to consider LGBT issues – especially connected to health – as transnational phenomena that are interconnected with local practices and meanings.

As stated by Ann Cvetkovich in *An Archive of Feeling: Trauma, Sexuality, and Lesbian Public Cultures*, queer archives "address particular versions of the determination to 'never forget' that gives archives of traumatic history their urgency" (Cvetkovich 2003: 242). Even if any documentary or visual product, as any other cultural object, is not a neutral product and further research is needed to interpret Hildebrand's gaze, the Face of AIDS film archive consists of assemblages of desires, experiences, narratives, and accounts, depictions of political conditions and individual resistance that challenge the coherence of a (single) narrative. Following Cvetkovich, Hildebrand's project is not aimed to search for "what really happened" or "what is really happening," neither is it "linearly structured around canonical events" (Edenheim 2013) but provides the chance to pay attention to ephemeral events and fragments that both give the archive a sense of urgency and deeply challenge the normative order (related to standardized form of expression, to plot construction and definition, to the expected audience, and to the values at stake).

While HIV- or AIDS-affected individuals are telling their stories they are at the same time offering potential listeners the chance to recognize what has been said. They are proffering a political statement and claiming social and sexual justice. As Boltanski stated, societies can offer two main kinds of reactions to suffering: the politics of pity and the politics of justice (Boltanski 1999). Interviews by Hildebrand do not focus merely on the pietistic aspects of their health status but ask the listener to consider the iniquities and structural disadvantages we are all forced to face. In particular, the gay population, the main subject of this chapter, offers their own biographies to the listeners: in this case, we all risk imprudently to "blame the victim" – as many of the same individuals with HIV from vulnerable groups because of their social class, ethnicity/race, or gender identity usually do blame themselves.

The action of blaming someone (or himself/herself) contributes to the eradication of an event from its political or economic context and the construction of victim hierarchies where someone is more of a victim than somebody else. Within this stratification of bodies, people living with HIV or AIDS usually blame just themselves. Stories of HIV, especially in developing countries, are often narratives of poverty, social exclusion, discrimination, corruption, insecurity, emergency, or broken families because of the exploitation of labor force, housing problems, stigmatization, religious persecution, ghetto or favela segregation, unavailability of antiretroviral drugs, and governmental unwillingness to provide treatments or implement health policies. Every story has a deep political meaning since it witnesses the misrecognition faced by bodies of nonnormative sexualities and *poz* bodies, targets of everyday and routinized violence (Scheper-Hughes 1992) and of political and structural violence (Farmer 2001; 2004). Those are *bodies who remember* (Fassin 2007).

Much of Staffan Hildebrand's archive related to the gay male population, specifically in developing countries, highlights the vulnerability of gay people living with HIV/AIDS or exposed to a high risk of virus transmission because of the structural, interpersonal, and symbolic violence they face.

These reflections will be clearer if we take into account the words of Gracia Violeta Ross Quiroga, HIV ambassador for Tearfund and campaigner for the rights of people living with HIV, who was interviewed in 2008 in Bolivia, when she was asked "Who are the people today that are getting infected from HIV?":

> The people who are getting infected in Bolivia with HIV are still a lot of the most vulnerable groups: men who have sex with men, young people, people living in the margins of the Bolivian society, and women. For a while we did not see so many cases of women and now this is going up very fast … and right now we see people from the indigenous groups also joining the groups and we are aware of some people who died of AIDS in the rural area [concerned].… In Bolivia, in societies like for example El Alto, the city of El Alto, which is a city made of internal migration, the poorest rural area in Bolivia expulses people to the big cities so they came here.… You know coming from a rural area with a conservative culture to a big city in which sex is available sometimes for free for some of them is actually making them vulnerable, also these cities that are populated with a lot of people create the situation of vulnerability for people you know, you have more

workers offering their services and less opportunities for all of them.... These people are highly vulnerable to HIV because they do not have information they face a new way of living and they also live in poor conditions and they do not have health insurance and for them living in big cities is very expensive.... We know migrant women face violence, women from indigenous groups are raped in the cities and not in their rural villages, and we are not addressing this properly in Bolivia.... I cannot tell a woman in El Alto ... use a condom and be safe, she cannot say this to her husband, if she says these words she will be beaten and she will face domestic violence and maybe will be killed. So, for these kinds of women I need other kind of messages.

(Archive ID: 2008_14_01)

Social suffering, personal experience of pain and suffering, as Ross Quiroga states, is usually imposed socially and structurally across race, class, gender, sexuality, and other power-ridden categories. Abusive relations, such as those implied in the stigmatization of people living with HIV, can be better understood as structured phenomena that encompass both structural and personal levels of analysis. Marginality and stigmatization related to HIV status are deeply connected, for example, to the lifestyle of the people involved, their social class and status, their housing condition, their presence or expulsion from the labor market, their eventual contacts with drug underworlds or the bureaucracies of social services and social control, their migrant or refugee status, their gender and gender role's codes.

To this end, since this volume is the product of contributors from different cultural backgrounds we do not intend to take for granted the still existing

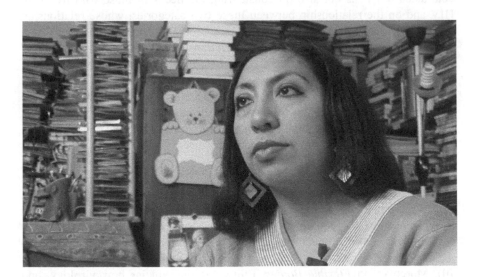

Figure 9.1 Gracia Violeta Ross Quiroga.
Source: Archive ID 2008_14_01.

stereotyped relation between homosexuality and AIDS. Instead, we will attempt to summarize the main sociological approaches that acknowledge the link that exists between AIDS and the stigmatization of nonnormative sexual conducts and then we will address the issue of structural violence and how it can be discerned in the impact of HIV/AIDS on oppressed and marginalized groups on a global scale, as manifested in the Face of AIDS film archive.

AIDS-homosexuality: how to construct a cultural enemy

The epidemic that resulted from the transmission of the HIV virus, despite being based on characteristically medical reflections at first, enabled the coexistence of pluralistic and diverse disciplinary narratives. These range from bio-psycho-medical theories to anthropological (ten Brummelhuis and Herdt 1995) and sociological (Nelkin, Willis, and Parris 1991) contributions; socioeconomic reflections linked (Bonnel *et al.* 2013), for example, to public health policies and measures in terms of global education policies (Wiseman and Glover 2012) and social action (Cannon Poindexter 2010); reflections on human rights (Correa, Petchesky and Parker 2008), and thoughts of a cultural (Rödlach 2006; Barz and Cohen 2011) and even artistic-literary (Subero 2013; 2014) and religious nature (Long 2005). These characteristics make AIDS a "total social fact," whose analysis enables researchers to interpret apparently unrelated phenomena, from health care policies and sexual rights to new forms of identity categorization and couple formation (serodiscordance).

In particular, we can see how over time HIV and AIDS, having become a transnational phenomenon, imposes a change of perspective in terms of individual health. The focus is no longer only on protecting those who have not yet contracted the virus but also on considering the needs of those who live with HIV and on the relationship between these two categories, whose relationship and intimacy are subject to forms of construction and categorization. HIV was not the first nor the only virus that took such transnational perspectives, but HIV/ AIDS was the first disease of globalization (Meruane 2014). Indeed,

> the decreasing cost of travel and the appearance of new communication technologies that had not been available to previous diseases were part of the long process of capitalism's structural and institutional transformation that began at the end of the nineteenth century.
>
> (Meruane 2014: 11)

Globalization helped both the disease to spread around the globe and, later on, it helped the treatments and medicine of the pharmaceutical companies to easily travel from country to country. The virus was able to connect the most developed with the less developed countries in the world and for this reason, according to Altman, "AIDS is both a product and a cause of globalization" (Altman 2001: 70). Moreover, in *Flexible Bodies*, Emily Martin explains how virology, and therefore AIDS, can be used as a metaphor in order to understand the workings of contemporary society (Martin 1994).

The sociological reflection on HIV and AIDS is closely interconnected with the social representation of nonnormative sexualities and particularly of male homosexuality. More than any other STD, AIDS – as it is associated not only with excess and sexual promiscuity regarded as "perversion" – turns the individual who contracts the virus by means of their sexual practices into a subject that is even more accountable for their own actions and "vices," and, consequently, even more worthy of blame. AIDS and the fears associated with it contribute to the construction of a specific social-sexual class that is seen as "dangerous" and "perverted," and which at the same time becomes the marker of an identity that can no longer be concealed. The AIDS epidemic and its *spectacularization* are proof of how the medical and political paranoia related to protecting the public space found in the homosexual subject the most appropriate scapegoat to protect the domestic and family dimension and to wage a conservative war against nonheteronormative sexualities, by strengthening monogamy, white sex, and "vanilla sex," reproduction and procreation within the context of marriage. The exacerbation of the stigma associated with both sexual orientation and health condition has contributed to link the threat of homosexuality to the fear of AIDS and contagion.

In the earliest stages of the epidemic gay men were immediately considered a high-risk group compared to the population as a whole. GRID (gay-related immune dysfunction) was the first invented acronym that constructed the gay community as the *exclusive* group affected and AIDS as a mainly *gay-related-disease*. The mischaracterization of AIDS as the "gay plight" and as a specific homosexual disease did not prevent heterosexuals from being involved in risky sexual behaviors. Fear of AIDS has affected social relations but also institutional and legal measures that have profoundly threatened LGBT people's rights during the AIDS crisis in terms of employment, housing, and freedom to travel but also in medical care, through discriminatory practices by insurance companies, the banning of gay bathhouses and bars and the proposal to quarantine or isolate AIDS patients, compulsory HIV testing for certain occupations (such as federal employees), and the banning of blood donation.

If, on the one hand, the AIDS epidemic brings the homosexual man back to the realm of abjection (Kristeva 1982), on the other hand it also allows subjects engaging in "bad sex" to acquire, because of the countless deaths and the marginalizing exposure to social stigma, a new sense of community. "Sexual perverts" and other marginalized subjects (drug users, sex workers, and black people) especially were able to denounce discrimination, to claim rights, and to develop solidarity networks revealing the intersections between many dimensions such as sexuality, social class, and race. The crisis related to AIDS and its public representation discredited the rehabilitation of the image of homosexuality, especially in contexts, such as the US one, where neoconservative governments were gaining ground. These instances brought about a renewal in gay and lesbian claims – radical movements that had homosexual ethnic minorities and sex rebels among them demanded a critical approach that was also geared toward broader institutional and cultural change. This led to not only the emergence of AIDS activists' organizations such as ACT UP (AIDS Coalition to Unleash Power), founded in New York in 1987, or Queer Nation and several other social change and advocacy groups but also the development of antinormative approaches such as queer theory (Seidman 1997).

The collected footage in the Face of AIDS film archive can also be discussed and interpreted in order to consider how these cultural repertoires take into account social inequalities which cause social suffering and affect specific individuals or groups in vulnerable status.

We will interpret our data, the footage in the archive, as evidence of *structural, interpersonal*, and *symbolic violence* faced by LGBT individuals. Violence actually operates along a continuum from structural violence (Farmer 2004; Scheper-Hughes and Bourgois 2004) to physical violence (such as direct homophobic assaults) and symbolic violence and everyday routinized violence (the imposition of the language and values of the dominant class, such as an ideology that naturalizes the hierarchies and subordination).

In particular, symbolic violence is a kind of violence which is exercised upon a social agent with his or her complicity (consider internalized homophobia, which can be regarded as deeply connected to the individual when they blames themselves or consider the "cultural silence" owing to rigid gender codes and gender role models within Latinos or African American communities), including structural violence hidden by hegemonic structures (such as governments, states or "globalized hegemonies") implemented by interventions and acts considered "moral" in the interests of hegemonic values ("extermination of the gay plague"). Structural violence is exerted *indirectly* and *systematically* by everyone who belongs to a specific social order, so when we deal with structural violence we must take into account all the dimensions in which oppression can occur. Consequently, every specific context is characterized by distinct structural circumstances. While some gay men – especially white – in developed countries have access to the labor market and are integrated somehow to the wage economy to get financial autonomy and independence from their families' household, many LGBTs in developing countries are precluded from independence from family and kin networks or lack access to education, to housing, or to the health care system and run a high risk of social exclusion if they deviate from normative sexual cultures.

LGBT ethnic minorities and specific segments of the population (such as black people or transgender individuals and sex workers) in industrialized societies and in developing countries could occupy a disadvantaged status because of social exclusion, stigmatization, and governmental policing undermining LGBT human rights. Social and medical anthropologists have demonstrated that rejection, stigmatization, or physical violence can contribute to further marginalization of LGBT people, especially when they lose support of social networks they use for survival, with worsened health conditions as a consequence.

To exemplify this violence, we used some materials of the Face of AIDS film archive. We started our research with the selection of one of the "key populations" available, the category of "Men Who Have Sex With Men." A total of fifty-three videos were present under this category; we decided not to consider four videos because two were documentaries made by Hildebrand and the other two were shots of panels at an International AIDS Conference. We watched the forty-nine videos left, of which nineteen were from "level 1," fifteen from "level 2," and fifteen from "level 3," which for privacy reasons were available only at Karolinska Institutet Library. Even if all the videos we watched gave us the opportunity to reflect and to draw our attention to both marginalized and vulnerable groups, at the end we chose to include in this chapter quotes from a total of ten videos, four from "level 1," three from "level 2," and three from "level 3." We included these videos because they offered the best examples of structural violence.

Social suffering and structural violence in the HIV epidemic

As previously mentioned, violence can operate simultaneously in structural, symbolic, personal, and intimate dimensions (Bourgois 1995; Scheper-Hughes and Bourgois 2004; Padilla, Vasquez del Aguila, and Parker 2007). In particular, Pierre Bourdieu's concept of symbolic violence can be useful to analyze the way practices link feeling to a social domination. Dominated and subordinated people misrecognize social inequalities as "the natural order" and blame themselves for their social conditions, using the same language of the dominants and thereby reproducing preconsciously the same hierarchies: in this way, social hierarchies are legitimized and naturalized (Bourdieu 1990; 2001). The analysis of social suffering and symbolic violence can be an effective tool to critique discrimination, stigmatization, and poverty in the case of HIV in vulnerable groups (because of their race, social class, and social status). This is particularly the case when such conditions are considered to be caused primarily by the victims themselves, because of their personal characteristics and behaviors. Taking into account Michel Foucault's concept of biopower as a form of governmentality (Foucault 2002; 2003), we could also pay attention to the way structurally imposed social suffering can produce destructive subjectivities – such as sex workers and those who are drug-addicted, for example – which are *lumpenized* or made more vulnerable because of their marginalized status. Some auto-destructive identities and conducts are forms of subjectification that emerge when biopower as a form of governmentality is internalized by neoliberal citizens (Bourgois 1995; 2009) or when states and governments do not grant human rights. A 32-year-old guy living with HIV since 1997 states in an interview from the Face of AIDS film archive that: "When you are poor you ... do certain behavior that you wouldn't if you would not poverty stricken and because you indulge in those behavior you put yourself in risk" (Archive ID: 2006_20_02).

Within developing countries the main concerns are related to the "cultural silence" of some ethnic-racial minorities or within specific cultural contexts where homosexual conduct is highly stigmatized such as among Latinos or the African American population in the United States (Diaz 1998). As stated by activist Martin Delaney in the Castro district in San Francisco, interviewed by Hildebrand:

> AIDS has moved in this city as has in so many to other regions, it is now in the black community, it is in the Latino community, it is in the tender line here where people use drugs, wherever there is poverty you will find AIDS that mingle with it.
>
> (Archive ID: 1998_7_04)

Those are the same communities that are at high risk of exposure to violence within their own ethnic group and to vulnerability compared to the wider society; they face both rejection from their families and group because of their sexual orientation or gender identity and discrimination from the white gay communities. Those are risk factors that together with other structural conditions – such as poverty, racism, social exclusion, discrimination, and criminalization – have a big impact on HIV risk behavior and other problems such as anger, low esteem, depression, drugs, and substance abuse (Diaz 1998; Hoppe 2017).

Phil Wilson, founder of the Black AIDS Institute in Los Angeles, states in another interview that:

> Among black gay men in America we definitely have a generalized epidemic, where we see incidence as high as 46% and prevalence as high as nearly 50% as well. A black gay man in America may very well be the most vulnerable population on the planet, clearly the most vulnerable population in the developed world and we have epidemic among black gay men in America that levels we see in the developing world in South Africa, in Botswana, in Zimbabwe, and elsewhere.

When Hildebrand asks "Why it is so difficult to approach this part of the epidemic in the black young gay men?" Wilson continues:

> I think that the fact in the United States we have a large epidemic and we have a complicated epidemic, we have an epidemic where we have to deal with social economic issues, where we have to deal with educational issues, where we have to deal with an uneven health delivery system, the fact that we have over 30 million Americans who do not have health care right now is a contributing factor to the spread of HIV in our community, it is the fact that for far too long some of the easy interventions were prohibited or difficult.
>
> (Archive ID: 2012_106)

High HIV risk behavior and transmission can also be associated with institutionalized homophobia and symbolic violence that lead individuals to internalize heterosexist values. This is what happened, for example, in Mexico or Bolivia among men who have sex with men, where rigid gender roles contribute to hide any connection to "polluted" homosexuality. In those countries, as AIDS activist Ricardo Baruch explains, society highly stigmatizes some sexual practices if they are performed by men (to be bottom) because of structural "machismo" and sexism (see Archive ID: 2007_25_01).

There exists a rigid gender role dichotomy and gender codes that also affect the definition of (male) hierarchies based on the dominance of the active (male) over the passive/receptive (feminized) one. These processes prompt close reflection on normative constructions of racialized masculinity, on the identification of the participants in the case, for example, of sex tourism (both sex workers and clients), and on the construction of male desire and pleasure. In this social order, gender lines and the sexuality of the body guarantee the cohesion of society: any attempt to destabilize this order is therefore a threat and a danger that must be avoided. The stratification of desire, especially of the white sex tourist and the indigenous middle and upper-middle classes, leads to the eroticization of the body and the physical characteristics associated with the working and lower classes. In saunas and public baths or in public sex venues and "cruising" areas masculine young men who come from rural areas are largely preferred and are in the highest demand (Rinaldi 2016). Such bodies are associated with virile and heterosexual masculinity, belonging to those who do not "feel pleasure" but do it because of necessity, not for emotional reasons but being part of the *trade*. Moreover, they are constantly put under pressure to ejaculate, as often requested by the client, which increases the price of the service and often leads to sex workers using drugs or accepting to perform unsafe sex practices.

In more structural terms, there are nations where there exist open interventions and policies to moralize (homo)sexual conduct and where homophobia is

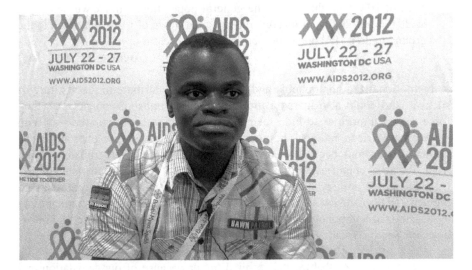

Figure 9.2 Paul Nsubuga Semugoma.
Source: Archive ID 2012_105.

state-sponsored, as Paul Nsubuga Semugoma from the Global Forum explains referring to Uganda, in response to a question about why homophobia is so strong in Uganda:

> It is a confluence of many issues.... Uganda has tended also to have quite a big influx of influence from the West, especially from America, from the US mainly missionaries, preachers who are on the right side of the American politics and thus anti-gay and kind of exports that bring that view to Ugandans. Ugandans are very religious and they tend to think because they are religious they cannot accept homosexuality. And also, the fact that gay people in Uganda are also a political scapegoat, an easy political scapegoat.

When asked about what can be done against homophobia, Nsubuga Semugoma continues:

> We have our neighbors, Kenya, for example which has the same laws currently on the books, which is the same because we are former British colonies, ok, similarly to Tanzania, but in Uganda we have tended to be more homophobic and less likely to take on these groups, the LGBT groups, the Men Who Have Sex With Men groups, whereas in Kenya with the same laws they are still able to take them, to measure this HIV prevention in those countries, and HIV prevention and care in those countries, now we are not doing it in Uganda because we say because of the laws but that is an excuse. Speaking from the point of fact that HIV is a big issue in the country, that we still have a generalized epidemic, that still more people are getting infected, that we have these groups which have actually documented high rates of HIV than the rest of the general population. I think we better put aside this, our high moralization, and just get down of it and get down to the ground to do it HIV prevention because it is necessary.
>
> (Archive ID: 2012_105)

Institutionalized homophobia and antigay laws contribute to the "culture of silence" and could also increase the risk of virus transmission because they force sexual minorities to hide themselves. In the case of Uganda – as with some other African nations – homophobia is strong in interpersonal and institutional dimensions because of the influence of religious integralism coming from Western countries through missionaries; as a former British colony, Uganda passed antigay laws that prevent policies and health treatments to prevent AIDS diffusion. It is the same in other African nations characterized by legitimized homophobia and instable governments, as in the case of Zimbabwe and South Africa:

> To be gay in Zimbabwe it is a bit difficult because of our legislation and also because our culture it is taboo in our culture.... In Zimbabwe or in South Africa our culture is almost intertwined, they are the same ... we went

also through the same process of denial, objections, stigma. In Zimbabwe, there is political instability.

> (Luiz from GALZ – Gays and Lesbians of Zimbabwe – in Archive ID:
> 2009_16_03)

There could also be examples of intergenerational violence within both developed and developing countries especially regarding children and young people who could be forced by adults to engage in sexual transactions or who engage in sex work or other sex in gay-identified "cruising" areas, situations that can increase risk to HIV exposure. This can also be true if we consider young people forced to leave their families and community because of their sexual orientation. Furthermore, young homeless people are usually subordinated by adults and engage as runaways in survival sex or in sexual tourism.

These are the main fears expressed by Tony Lisle, UNAIDS country coordinator in Cambodia, in the following interview:

> There is clear evidence that males having sex with males who are discovered by their families, there are instances where they are kicked out by their families, they are often on the streets, they often then reverted to selling sex to survive.
>
> HILDEBRAND: What you say about these teenage boys selling sex, it is something that increasing in Cambodia or what have got to do with the epidemic?
> LISLE: I think sex work overall, and particularly indirect sex work and transactional sex, whether these are young people, young women or young men is definitely increasing. We see a move away from brothel buy sex to non-brothel buy sex.
> HILDEBRAND: How do you describe these teenage boys?
> LISLE: Many of these young boys selling sex because they there is an economic imperative, they are poor, they have very few employment opportunities, and so they are pushed to selling sex, to transactional sex.
>
> (Archive ID: 2007_5_02)

Sex workers can also face violence from passersby and discrimination by governmental forces such as police who can discipline people involved in sex in public settings.

Classed and generational violence is not just a characteristic of poor non-industrialized nations. Larry Kramer, AIDS activist and playwright, interviewed by Hildebrand, confessed that it was like a brotherhood genocide:

> I murdered people, I made a list of all the people I slept with between 1981 and 19 whatever was when the drugs came, no! Until the virus was discovered that's it, five years I slept with over hundreds of people and I looked down that list of how many of them have died and a lot of them died and

probably I murdered much of them you know the kids I fucked for the first time in their life whatever. You have to think in those terms that we have murdered each other, our own brothers, and no one talks like that and we have to talk like that. That is the only way people will behave better I hope, I don't know.

(Archive ID: 2006_1)

A patient dying from AIDS at San Francisco General Hospital in 1988 expressed the same fear and blamed classed and generational structural violence in the following exchange:

I still have a little bit of fear of having sex with someone because I do not want to infect anyone, I find that if I do have sex with someone it is, involves love more, it involves me feeling for them and it involves me being aware they can feel for me.

HILDEBRAND: What do you have to say to a boy of 15/16 that he is selling himself for money today to the men?
THE PATIENT: If you have to sell yourself if the necessity is there if you are not going to any of the support groups that can get you out of that remember safe sex, remember you can be paid more for not using a condom but whoever is paying you that more is taking away your life.

(Archive ID: 1988_189)

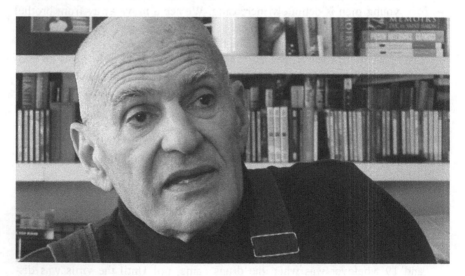

Figure 9.3 Larry Kramer.
Source: Archive ID 2006_1.

For a conclusion: trauma and social suffering

Hildebrand's main contribution is to have framed HIV and AIDS as a global phenomenon that gave us the opportunity of not only taking into account culture-specific gay subjectivation but also their particular biographical accounts. This has provided a global vision that forces Western individuals to consider other forms of gender construction and (homo)sexualities that differ profoundly from normative white, masculine, status privileged Western (US and EU) models (Oswin 2006). The work of Hilbedrand can also be useful to question several issues, among which, for example, HIV-prevention models are usually constructed according to normative and Western categories that disadvantage some ethnic groups and nonnormative gender individuals.

This chapter has demonstrated that the Face of AIDS film archive can contribute to show how social inequalities cause social suffering in marginalized and vulnerable groups. Indeed, the Face of AIDS film archive is much more than a collection of footage of the last thirty years. It tells the stories of minorities but not as stories of pity or of blame. It represents the stories of resistance, courage, and the will to live and to help others in an unprecedented transnational way.

The work of Hildebrand is part of what Cvetkovich called queer archives and the urgency of never forgetting (Cvetkovich 2003). The people depicted in this footage ask us to be remembered, because we should never forget the HIV/AIDS pandemic.

As we presented in this text, HIV/AIDS is a total social fact. HIV/AIDS is a complex and multifaceted phenomenon that needs specific forms of intervention, especially when marginalized and vulnerable groups are involved. The sense of community among these groups was pivotal in the fight against the disease. Indeed, in the general culture of silence, it was only thanks to this new sense of community that arose in the 1980s that homosexual people were able to survive. Only when this wall of silence was broken the first medical solutions were found. But the fight is not over yet. On the one hand, developing countries need our attention because, as we wrote in these pages, the prevalence of HIV is still surprisingly high and, on the other hand, in developed countries an increasing number of people have the feeling that HIV has been defeated and are now engaging in risky sexual practices abandoned more than thirty years ago.

Moreover, further research must take into account the way in which documentarism can create *othered* global subjectivities and how in the visual imagery of the filmmaker (or the journalist) and in the people represented race, gender, sexual orientation, social class, and able-bodiedness still intersect and structure inequality. In this way the filmmaker – especially in this case – becomes a cultural producer who implicitly contributes to the collection and recording of collective trauma archives: viewing the gay epidemic in a global visual setting provides vulnerable subjectivities the chance to resist normative order and to challenge oppression systems.

Note

1 This chapter has been discussed by both authors. However, Marco Bacio authored the sections titled "AIDS-homosexuality: how to construct a cultural enemy" and "For a conclusion. Trauma and social suffering," while Cirus Rinaldi authored the sections titled "Introduction. Structural and symbolic violence and LGBT issues – a transnational phenomenon" and "Social suffering and structural violence in the HIV epidemic."

References

Altman, Dennis (2001), *Global Sex*. Chicago, IL: University of Chicago Press.

Barz, Gregory and Judah M. Cohen, eds. (2011). *The Culture of Aids in Africa: Hope and Healing in Music and the Arts*. Oxford: Oxford University Press.

Boltanski, Luc (1999). *Distant Suffering: Morality, Media and Politics*. Cambridge: Cambridge University Press.

Bonnel, René, Rosalía Rodriguez-Garcia, Jill Olivier, Quentin Wodon, Sam McPherson, Kevin Orr, and Julia Ross (2013). *Funding Mechanisms for Civil Society: The Experience of the AIDS Response*. Washington, DC: The World Bank.

Bourdieu, Pierre (1990). *The Logic of Practice*. Cambridge: Polity Press in association with Basil Blackwell.

Bourdieu, Pierre (2001). *Masculine Domination*. Stanford, CA: Stanford University Press.

Bourgois, Philippe I. (1995). *In Search of Respect: Selling Crack in El Barrio*. New York: Cambridge University Press.

Bourgois, Philippe I. and Jeff Schonberg, (2009). *Righteous Dopefiend*. Berkeley, CA: University of California Press.

Cannon Poindexter, Cynthia, ed. (2010). *Handbook of HIV and Social Work: Principles, Practice, and Populations*. Hoboken, NJ: John Wiley & Sons.

Corrêa, Sonia, Rosalind Petchesky, and Richard Parker (2008). *Sexuality, Health and Human Rights*. London and New York: Routledge.

Cvetkovich, Ann (2003). *An Archive of Feelings: Trauma, Sexuality, and Lesbian Public Cultures*. Durham, NC: Duke University Press.

Diaz, Rafael M. (1998). *Latino Gay Men and HIV*. London and New York: Routledge.

Edenheim, Sara (2013). "Lost and Never Found: The Queer Archive of Feelings and Its Historical Propriety," *Differences*, 24(3): 36–62.

Farmer, Paul (2001). *Infections and Inequalities*. Berkeley, CA: University of California Press.

Farmer, Paul (2004). "An Anthropology of Structural Violence," *Current Anthropology*, 45(3): 305–325.

Fassin, Didier (2007). *When Bodies Remember: Experiences and Politics of AIDS in South Africa*. Berkeley, CA: California University Press.

Foucault, Michel (2002). "The Subject and Power," in Michel Foucault, *Power: Essential Works of Foucault 1954–1984*, Volume 3. London: Penguin.

Foucault, Michel (2003). *Society Must Be Defended. Lecture Series at the Collège de France, 1975–76*. London: Penguin.

Hoppe, Trevor (2017). *Punishing Disease: HIV and the Criminalization of Sickness*. Oakland, CA: University of California Press.

Kristeva, Julia (1982). *Powers of Horror: An Essay on Abjection*. New York: Columbia University Press.

Long, Thomas L. (2005). *AIDS and American Apocalypticism: The Cultural Semiotics of an Epidemic.* Albany, NY: State University of New York Press.

Martin, Emily (1994). *Flexible Bodies: Tracking Immunity in American Culture from the Days of Polio to the Age of AIDS.* Boston, MA: Beacon Press.

Meruane, Lina (2014). *Viral Voyages. Tracing AIDS in Latin America.* New York: Palgrave Macmillan.

Nelkin, Dorothy, David P. Willis, and Scott V. Parris, eds. (1991). *A Disease of Society: Cultural and Institutional Responses to AIDS.* Cambridge: Cambridge University Press.

Oswin, Natalie (2006). "Decentering Queer Globalization: Diffusion and the 'Global Gay,'" *Environment and Planning D: Society and Space*, 24: 777–790.

Padilla, Mark B., Ernesto Vasquez del Aguila, and Richard G. Parker (2007). "Globalization, Structural Violence, and LGTB Health: A Cross-Cultural Perspective," in I. Meyer and M. Northridge (eds.), *The Sexual Health of Sexual Minorities. Public Health Perspectives on Lesbian, Gay, Bisexual and Transgender Health*, pp. 209–241. New York: Kluwer Academic/Plenum.

Parker, Richard (2002). "The Global HIV/AIDS Pandemic, Structural Inequalities, and the Politics of International Health," *Global HIV/AIDS*, 92(3): 343–346.

Rinaldi, Cirus (2016). "(Homosexual) Male Sex Work: Sociological Representations, Social Realities and New Normalizations," in F. Jacob (ed.), *Prostitution: Eine Begleiterin der Menschheit/a Companion of Mankind*, pp. 99–118. New York: Peter Lang.

Rödlach, Alexander (2006). *Witches, Westerners, and HIV: AIDS & Cultures of Blame in Africa.* Walnut Creek, CA: Left Coast Press.

Scheper-Hughes, Nancy (1992). *Death without Weeping: The Violence of Everyday Life in Brazil.* Berkeley, CA: University of California Press.

Scheper-Hughes, Nancy and Philippe Bourgois (2004). "Introduction: Making Sense of Violence," in N. Scheper-Hughes and P. Bourgois (eds.), *Violence in War and Peace.* Oxford: Blackwell, pp. 1–27.

Seidman, Steven (1997). *Difference Troubles: Queering Social Theory and Sexual Politics.* Cambridge: Cambridge University Press.

Subero, Gustavo, ed. (2013). *HIV in World Cultures: Three Decades of Representations.* New ed. London and New York: Routledge.

Subero, Gustavo (2014). *Representations of HIV/AIDS in Contemporary Hispano-American and Caribbean Culture. Cuerpos suiSIDAs.* Farnham: Ashgate.

ten Brummelhuis, Han and Herdt, Gilbert, eds. (1995). *Culture and Sexual Risk. Anthropological Perspectives on AIDS.* Amsterdam: Gordon and Breach.

Wiseman, Alexander W. and Ryan N. Glover, eds. (2012). *The Impact of Hiv/Aids on Education*, Volume 18. Bingley: Emerald.

10 Constructions of safe sex

Between desire and governmentality

Mariah Larsson

Introduction: how to have sex in an epidemic

In 1983, two gay men compiled what is probably the first booklet on safer sex techniques. *How to Have Sex in an Epidemic: One Approach* was written by Richard Berkowitz and Michael Callen under the consultation of Joseph Sonnabend, MD (Berkowitz and Callen 1983). In those first few years of the AIDS epidemic, before the HIV virus was identified, before anything was clear on how the mysterious disease actually transmitted, the "lifestyle" of the gay communities in San Francisco and New York had already become demonized and regarded as a cause and even origin of the strange immunodeficiency syndrome that seemed to afflict in particular young men who had sex with men.

Although the advice in the booklet takes as its point of departure a theory of the cause of AIDS that later was abandoned, and therefore actually restricts behavior slightly more than necessary (for instance, claiming that the virus can be transmitted by urine), it is basically sound advice for anyone who wants to attempt to have sex in a way that reduces the risk of passing on or contracting HIV or other sexually transmitted infections. Use a condom, avoid the exchange of bodily fluids, and try to swap contact info so that you can get in touch with your partner in case of an (any) STI.

The booklet was, in a way, a desperate attempt to do something in a situation where knowledge was scarce, a response to the question "should we stop having sex?" that tried to find a middle way between moral panic and denial. In the introduction, Berkowitz and Callen explain their view: "As you read on, we hope we make at least one point clear: Sex does not make you sick – diseases do. Gay sex does not make you sick – gay men who are sick do" (Berkowitz and Callen 1983: 3). Throughout the booklet, the significant point is that you, the reader, should continue to have sex as much as you want to. It is the particular ways you have sex that might be dangerous, not the sex itself. Nevertheless, the issue of sexual morals does resonate as an underlying tone. Toward the end of the booklet there is a discussion about love. "Without affection, it is less likely that you will care as much if you give your partner disease." Further on, they write, "Too many gay men get together for only two reasons: to exploit each other and to be exploited" (Berkowitz and Callen 1983: 38, 39). Accordingly, the booklet ends on a note that contradicts or at least qualifies the introductory message: on the one hand, you can have as much sex, in safe ways, as you want to, but on the other you should care about your sexual partners at least enough to not exploit them and not give them disease. The message of safe sex is thus infused with a message about emotional involvement and responsibility.

Ever since AIDS was first identified, the very discovery of the mysterious disease afflicting mainly young gay men was construed as connected to a "life-style," implicating bathhouses, promiscuity, anal sex, the use of poppers (which was even discussed as a possible cause in the beginning), and so on. The initial denomination of "GRID" (gay-related immune deficiency) specified a principal population (and thereby implying a specific lifestyle) rather than the disease itself (see e.g., Treichler 1999; Watney 1987; France 2016). Already at the point of its earliest discovery, HIV/AIDS was connected to behavior, lifestyle, and moral attitude, but also to issues of governmentality, sex education, individual responsibility, and public health policies.

In this chapter, I will argue that, although the conceptualization of safe (or safer) sex may seem morally neutral because it is based in medical fact, in reality it very rarely is. In addition, like the entire issue of HIV and AIDS, discussions and communication of safe sex practices unfold across the field of public and private. Safe sex is intertwined with questions about responsibility, sexual conduct, gender roles, and governmentality. By making various touchdowns in the Face of AIDS film archive, I will compare and discuss how HIV/AIDS and safer sex practices have been discursively constructed by physicians, research-ers, activists, educators, and people living with HIV or AIDS in 1988, 1998, and 2008 in various parts of the world: the Philippines, Australia, Sweden, the U.S., Thailand, Morocco, and Bolivia.

Theoretical perspectives

There are several theoretical concepts that inform the perspective of this study. Most significant are sociologists John H. Gagnon and William Simon's idea about sexual scripts and the Foucauldian notions about biopower and govern-mentality. Sexual script theory postulates that sexuality is socially constructed and describes how this works on three levels: the intrapsychic script (which is the individual's own fantasies and desires), the interpersonal script (governing what happens between two or more people), and the cultural scenario (provid-ing both a backdrop to and information for the other two levels) (Gagnon and Simon 2005). All three of these are relevant for the issue of safer sex practices as well as for the conceptualizations of safe sex: In order to be actually effec-tual, condom use and other sexual practices that decrease the risk of virus trans-mission need to be made into a part of the fabric of the intrapsychic sexual script so they can be employed at the interpersonal level (Gagnon and Simon 2005). In order for them to be incorporated into the intrapsychic sexual script, they need to be emphasized on the cultural level, both as information and as a something "sexy."

What is more, strategies for implementing safer sex within a national or global population quite logically, as others have observed, call to mind Foucauldian notions of governmentality and biopower (Foucault 1990). When the "AIDS scare" or "moral panic" was at its peak in the mid- to late 1980s (at the time when Hildebrand began his documentation), various proposals and suggestions, as well as actual legislative change, of a repressive and discriminatory kind were plentiful. One remarkable example from Sweden in 1986 was the proposal, published in a series of articles in the press by two physicians, that HIV testing should be compulsory and that people with HIV should be isolated from the rest of society (Tibbling 1987). The argument in the articles was, basically, that promiscuous homosexuality was "urge-driven," much like drug use, and individuals engaging in that kind of behavior could not be counted on to show consideration to other people (Tibbling 1987: 17, 34). As much as this proposal was met with outrage and angry replies (and never came to fruition), it is illustrative both of the heteronormative reaction to AIDS and of the notion of disciplining people's bodies, as well as of the prevailing sense of doom: desperate measures for desperate times, in order to protect the "good" people of society.

Nonetheless, already in 1985, Sweden had included HIV and AIDS in the Contagious Disease Act, meaning that individuals living with HIV were responsible for informing potential partners about their HIV status before engaging in sexual activity. The inclusion of the HIV virus in the Contagious Disease Act can be regarded as an attempt at making sex safer on a large-scale level and containing the spread of HIV, regardless of condom use, abstinence, sexual practices, or medication. Although this measure has been severely criticized as oppressive and counterproductive, both nationally (e.g., Henriksson and Ytterberg 1992) and internationally (e.g., Baldwin 2005; see Bredström 2008), it has also, from a public health perspective, been considered an unfortunate but reasonable and necessary way of controlling the disease (see Kallings 2005). On this large-scale level, the measures taken to control the spread of HIV and AIDS, regardless of their benevolence or malice, can be understood as expressions of biopower, as a way for the state to control the human body in order to limit the spread of a disease. However, and as we will see, the biopower exerted over the sexual mind is of no less significance but has less predictable outcomes.

Safer sex, sexual practices, and moral attitudes

Early on in the epidemic, knowledge came to be seen as a key element in preventive work. Although HIV/AIDS have been said by some to humble physicians and medical scientists, who thought they were on the way to solving everything (cf. Archive ID: 1988_147), it was also in a sense a triumph for enlightenment: sex education, controversial in many places, was quickly recognized as vital in the struggle against HIV/AIDS, although there was disagreement as to what this sex education should teach. However, education in itself was not enough; it was hoped to lead to a change in attitudes and, consequently, a change in behavior. Just knowing that a condom will protect you does not necessarily mean that you will accept condom use and actually use the condom in a sexual situation. Therefore, information was combined with moral, ethical, logical, and emotional arguments to bring forth a change in attitude.

Accordingly, tracing the various discourses around safe sex, safer sex, and unsafe sex that emerge in interviews with different subjects in the Face of AIDS film archive at different points in time will provide a historical and geographically diverse perspective on notions of morality. Owing to space and time limitations, only a few samples from the archive will be discussed, but this study can be regarded as a qualitative pilot study that only purports to point out some examples of how these discourses of morality may take shape. I have used the search terms "safe sex," "unsafe sex," and "safer sex" and chosen to focus on three different points in time, thus filtering the results by narrowing them to 1988, 1998, and 2008. These years are evenly spaced at ten-year intervals and each of them also represents a different phase in the global history of HIV/AIDS. For each time period, the choice of geographical place has been determined by which locations have been available, but I wanted a wide spread across the globe for each year. Also, I wanted different kinds of interviewees. In the final selection, there is one virologist at the center of the global mobilization against HIV/AIDS, one high school teacher, one social worker, two young men, one politician, one representative of a sex education organization, one young physician, and some activists. The clips are very different, in content, in duration, in context, and in subject. For each clip, I posed the questions: How is safe sex defined? Who or what is identified as a threat or the enemy? Where is responsibility placed? I have not been interested in the representativeness of the clips – that is, for instance, I will not draw any conclusions from the interview with Mechai Viravaidya in Thailand in 1998 as to how Thailand regarded safe sex in general. Rather, I will try to draw a kind of sketchy map of different approaches to and constructions of safe sex by the people being interviewed.

The first is 1988, when the Face of AIDS project was begun in earnest. The HIV virus was identified and the process from transmission to fully developed immunodeficiency was lined out. There were various attempts at treating the virus, and much experimentation in order to find a vaccine and/or a cure. In addition, and perhaps most importantly, in 1988 AIDS was no longer regarded as a phenomenon isolated to the gay population as it seemed to threaten the general, straight population, which in turn led to an "AIDS scare" or "AIDS panic" (Månsson and Hilte, 1990). When Hildebrand embarked on his project to document the HIV/AIDS epidemic, there was a strongly felt fear among educators, public health people, and physicians as well as the general community that AIDS would perhaps even wipe out humankind. Here, I have selected one clip from Sweden, two from the Philippines, and one from Australia.

By 1998, antiretroviral treatment was available in developed countries and the focus of the threat of HIV/AIDS had moved from the Western world to the African and Asian continents. In many Western countries, the panic had subsided and, consequently, information campaigns and educational ventures decreased. However, the available treatment was very expensive, which further reinforced already existing unequal economic power balances, both within nations like the U.S. and between nations across the world. This is also the year when the number of new HIV infections began to decline (https://timeline.avert. org/?129/AIDS-related-deaths-fall). For 1998, I have selected two clips from the U.S.A. and two from Thailand.

In 2008, the situation had stabilized. In the U.S., recommendations had been issued for postexposure prophylaxis in 2005. Preexposure prophylaxis would not be approved of until 2014, however. The high point of new HIV infections as well as of AIDS-related deaths had passed (https://ourworldindata.org/hiv-aids). Still, however, the HIV and AIDS issue highlights global inequality, gender imbalances, educational levels, and health policies. HIV/AIDS has been pushed to the background in people's minds, as has the question of safer sex. Here, I have chosen one clip from Sweden, another one from Bolivia, and a third, shot at the Seventeenth International AIDS Conference, in Mexico City, in which a young physician from Morocco is interviewed.

A commonly suggested strategy by scientists and educators, throughout, is education. This is most heavily emphasized in the clips from 1988, but the issue is present in the 1998 and 2008 clips as well. As long as there were no vaccines, no cure, and not even a functional way to halt the progress of the virus in the human blood, behavioral changes based on knowledge of how HIV is transmitted (for instance, consistent use of condoms) were actually the only way to prevent the epidemic. In two of the selected clips from 1988, both the Swedish physician and the Philippine teacher stress, although in different ways, the importance of knowledge and education, whereas in the one from Australia information is passed on in a very specific and succinct manner. However, although the situation for treatment has improved in 1998 and 2008, there is still no vaccine and education remains the most significant method to avoid the spread of HIV. In one of the clips from 2008, the Swedish interviewee actually says that one reason for Sweden having a comparatively low prevalence of HIV is the strong tradition of sex education in schools.

1988: "nature is bigger than mankind"

Dr. Lars Olof Kallings, from Statens Bakterologiska Laboratorium, draws upon metaphors of warfare and describes the HIV virus as a "clever enemy" that hides in the body (1988_147). To battle this enemy, scientists all over the world have mobilized. Another significant element in this battle is knowledge, and after having watched the repeated retakes of the thirty-six-minute clip I can only assume that the strongest motivation for Kallings to participate in Hildebrand's film was to spread that knowledge, because he does not seem entirely comfortable in front of the camera. When Hildebrand asks him to make a movement to adjust the focus in the microscope again, he responds, "Do I have to?" before he complies. Again and again, he scrupulously details what we know about how the virus transmits, and he seems extremely conscientious.

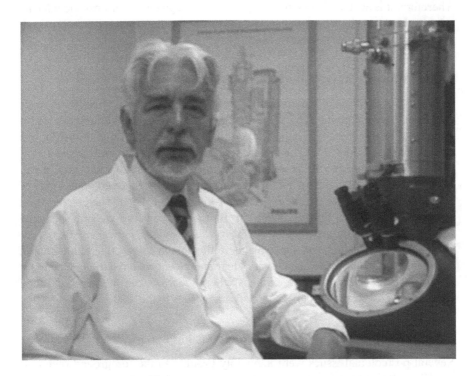

Figure 10.1 Lars Olof Kallings.
Source: Archive ID 1988_47.

At one point, he says that AIDS research has forced scientists to "look into dark corners" and that AIDS can be seen as a "torch lighting up dark corners in society." Probed by Hildebrand, he qualifies this evocative pronouncement: by "dark corners" he means drug addiction, a lack of social security and health insurance, and a deficient system of primary health care. Although he emphasizes knowledge as the only way to prevent HIV, he also explains that an upgrade of the health sector is of outmost importance. Kallings is reluctant to speak about issues outside his area of expertise but, prompted by Hildebrand, he says that, philosophically, AIDS could be seen as a message from nature that has to do with changes in lifestyle: global communications, traveling, world trade, and drug addiction are all part of the modern world and have contributed to the spread of the virus. When Hildebrand asks him about "true love," he chooses instead to use a slogan from Uganda: "love carefully."

As a physician and as involved in the global struggle against AIDS, Kallings can be said to have a macro perspective on the spread of the virus. His point of view is not on a national, regional, or individual level but on an international scale. For him, the concept of safe or safer sex must necessarily be only one weapon against AIDS, but at this point in time it is also the only one available.

Therefore, it is absolutely essential to get this message out, to inform and educate people about how to protect themselves, not only for their own sakes but, in fact, for the greater good of humanity.

1988: "what we have to do is be more specific"

In a brief scene, a social worker at the Australian Prostitutes Collective answers questions over the phone. The scene is very short, not even five minutes, and it begins with the camera moving toward a house and entering through the door as the phone rings (1988_21). The female social worker picks up and begins a conversation with someone on the other end of the line. From what she says, it can be surmized that the caller is a married man who is worried about what kinds of sex he can have with sex workers without risking transmission. The conversation is cut off before it is finished when the film scene ends, so we only hear the information about oral sex that the social worker provides. However, she is very calm and matter-of-fact, and she explains to the person calling that talking about "exchange of bodily fluids" is not very clear and "what we have to do is be more specific there." Succinctly, she explains where the virus can be found and why performing oral sex on a man can be very dangerous to the "lady."

1988: "so much damage western societies have made"

Several postcolonial issues were inevitably brought to the foreground owing to the HIV/AIDS epidemic. Residues of colonial pasts became acutely apparent in the global AIDS crisis – not least because issues of sexuality, gender equality, educational opportunities, and economic growth performed a vital role in how the responses to the threat played out. When asked whether "western values have infected" the Philippines, Eddy the teacher responds that there is "so much damage western societies have done," in a statement that most likely refers to the situation of HIV/AIDS and yet echoes of a long history of Western presence on the Philippine islands (1988_79). However, as the interview progresses, it is quite clear that by "Western" Eddy means American or Anglo-American ("rock culture" and "Hollywood" being explicitly pointed out as causes of changed values in Philippine society), and not the Catholicism inherited from 300 years of Spanish rule. In several clips from a Philippine Catholic school, Eddy is interviewed by Hildebrand and is shown teaching sex education to his students, and the students are interviewed about love, sex, and AIDS. The two clips I use here are of the interview with Eddy and from his sex education class.

Eddy is passionate and articulate: Sexual liberalism spreads AIDS and Western values have made traditional family values obsolete. Young people are abandoned and look to idols from rock music and Hollywood movies, which makes them out of touch with reality. The government should launch a massive sex education campaign but are afflicted with "bureaucratic inertia" and suppress vital information because they are worried that the tourism industry will be damaged by the AIDS crisis. Prostitution comes out of poverty because poor people have little choice (1988_79). In class, he states authoritatively that there are only two ways to protect yourself against AIDS: to use the condom and to have only one partner (1988_68).

1998: "check your lifestyle"

As the 1990s progressed, antiretroviral treatment became available, although it was a complex and expensive medication. In the two clips from the U.S. that I selected, issues of social difference are brought to the foreground by the young men being interviewed. Both of them, however, stress the importance of safer sex as the only way for the individual to protect him or herself. "You can't really trust someone," the young black man from the Bronx states (1998_5_06). "You don't know about their history." There seems to be a shift in the view of responsibility – using a condom and practicing safer sex is conceived of as taking care of yourself in a world where no one else cares.

Nonetheless, there are a number of differences between the way safe sex is conceptualized. The young black man from the Bronx – who seems to be older than the young Asian man in the other clip – has a more philosophical and wide-reaching view of sexuality and life in general: promiscuity and drugs are dangerous and you have to "check your lifestyle" to "reduce the risk." He includes a social analysis that brings in economic class difference as a significant element: "when you're poor, you're stressed out, you have no money" and that makes you "careless with the genitals." Protection has to become a "natural thing."

1998: "I think AIDS is like the Vietnamese war"

The other, younger man explains that you have to use condoms (1998_34_03). "My friends say it's better without the condom 'cause it's real sex but with the condom you're safe." When asked whether AIDS is a political issue, that rich people can get medicine that costs 30,000 dollars but poor people can't, he agrees and then goes on to state "just have safe sex or don't have sex at all," which he then modifies to "if you're married and have sex to have babies, but if you're just having sex for fun put on a condom." On the one hand, he seems to have an idea about the government as somehow accountable – because he says that "I think AIDS is like the Vietnamese war" – and on the other he points to the individual's responsibility, because "no one cares about us living or dying out here." In the face of the government's indifference, you have to take care of yourself.

1998: "if your mind is clean, the condom is not dirty"

Thailand's initial response of denial to the threat of HIV/AIDS was changed in the early 1990s into an active governmental campaign on several fronts to halt the spread of the virus. In both the clips I have selected, the agency of government and larger societal institutions is emphasized, in sharp contrast to the individual focus of the two American interviews. This might, obviously, be due to the fact that the American interviewees are representatives of the "common man" or "young Americans" in general, whereas the two people interviewed in Thailand have both been active within various organizations (including, for one of them, the government) attempting to stop the epidemic.

In a lengthy clip, Mechai Viravaidya, influential in several NGOs and NPOs, is interviewed about HIV and AIDS in Thailand. Viravaidya describes how a fear that information on HIV and AIDS would prove detrimental to tourism kept the government from doing anything in the late 1980s, but how, as he was appointed minister of tourism and information in 1991 (after the military coup), the government became very active in distributing HIV/AIDS information and educating people. "AIDS is not a medical problem, it is a behavioral problem. It does not only involve doctors and nurses but teachers, priest, taxi drivers – anyone who can change behavior and attitudes can be involved," Viravaidya says in the interview, going on to describe how education now begins in grades four to five, how information is spread on television and radio, at gas stations and through posters at bus stops (1998_10_01). "Thailand," he says, "was the first country in Asia to come out of the dark ages of denial." For Viravaidya, "the individual and the family was the core" to AIDS-prevention in the long term.

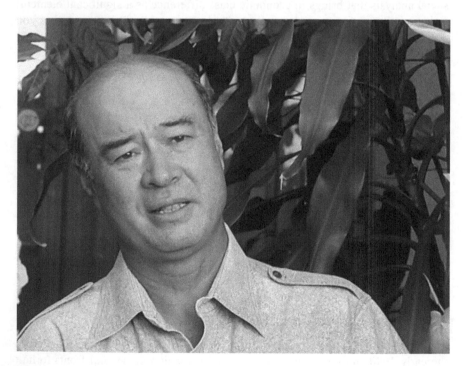

Figure 10.2 Mechai Viravaidya.
Source: Archive ID 1998_10_01.

1998: "AIDS is a two-edged sword"

The other Thai is a young activist. As Viravaidya has emphasized compassion as a weapon against AIDS, the activist observes that "AIDS is a two-edged sword," being devastating but also having taught him to be more human in a society where money-making has priority over the human aspects of life (1998_13_01). From his perspective, safe sex seems largely an issue of society and the government.

2008: "to convince people of the significance of condom use"

In the Swedish clip from 2008, Katarina Lindahl, who was at the time secretary general of the Swedish Association for Sexuality Education (RFSU), is interviewed for about seven minutes. At this point in time, retrospection had entered into the HIV and AIDS discourse, and much of the interview is about the past. Lindahl mentions people she has worked with and campaigns that were successful. In addition, she reflects on how Sweden has fared in relation to other parts of the world, and declares that the openness to talk about sexuality and the established sex education in schools has been very helpful in protecting people in Sweden with regards to HIV. When speaking about issues related to safer sex, she stresses that an important issue for today is to avoid HIV among young people. Considering the spread of chlamydia, she says, HIV would, given an entry point into that population, probably spread quite rapidly, too, and therefore good information campaigns are necessary, in which both organizations and authorities work together, using all the knowledge and experience that exist. The big challenge, she says, is to get the condom on, and when asked about what she wishes for the future she wishes for a really good way of convincing people about the significance of actually using the condom (2008_109_01).

2008: "gender inequality is one of the main drivers of this epidemic"

In the selected clip from Bolivia, gender inequality is pointed to as "one of the main drivers" of the HIV/AIDS epidemic by the two interviewed activists, Gracia Violeta Ross Quiroga and Juan Carlos Reja. Ross Quiroga eloquently explains that, by conforming to gender roles, men put themselves at risk and thereby also put the women at risk, because the male role does not acknowledge vulnerability (2008_13_01). Gender roles affect sexual behavior and risk behavior, and are thus not compatible with safer sex. Here, the problem does not originate with the government or the individual but rather at the level of a general and abstract ideological structure in society, a traditional machismo patriarchy that provides an untenable gender role for men because it does not include the conceptualization of men as possibly vulnerable. As women have less power in society, the male gender role puts her at risk as well.

2008: "this holistic approach is missing"

At the Seventeenth International AIDS Conference, in Mexico City, Staffan Hildebrand interviews a young physician from Morocco. Previously during the conference she has spoken out against the teaching of abstinence or even the "ABC" programs, that is, educational programs teaching to Abstain from sex, to Be faithful, and to use the Condom (2008_70_01). Hildebrand asks her to elaborate, and she explains that young people's sexual and reproductive lives are much more complicated, involving issues of responsibility, gender equality, loving, and caring, and cannot be summed up in "one letter, or three letters" (2008_70_02). Also, she states, "these programs have dramatically failed." Young people are having sex. Unwanted pregnancies and infections are going up, which could have been avoided with a more "holistic and comprehensive approach."

Discursive constructions of safe sex

An important aspect of the way safe sex is discussed and talked about in these clips is how they are framed and constructed as filmed interviews, and then indexed and archived in the Face of AIDS film archive. In all clips, Hildebrand asks questions that influence the answers. In some cases, Hildebrand is very persistent, like when he wants Kallings to talk about whether AIDS is a message from nature (1988_147) or when he asks the young Asian man to repeat his words about AIDS being like the Vietnamese War (1998_34_03). In others, he is more low-key. Depending on the microphone, his questions are not always

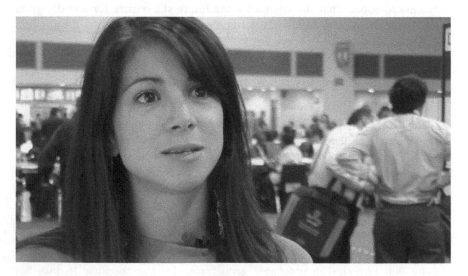

Figure 10.3 Imane Khachani.
Source: Archive ID 2008_70_02.

audible. However, there are certain themes that Hildebrand likes to touch upon: optimism, true love, hope. Obviously, the interviewer also affects the interviewee by providing supportive or disapproving gestures or facial expressions. Since Hildebrand is off camera, we cannot know whether he is an animated or passive interviewer, but the people being interviewed are not simply interacting with the camera or a presumed future spectator but foremost with Hildebrand and his cameraman.

Later, the archivists who indexed the clips to make them searchable had to interpret and classify the topics of the interviews. When I type in "safe sex" in the search box, the results reflect this process. In the clips I found and ultimately selected, safe sex is not necessarily an explicit subject but one aspect of everything the interviewed persons talk about. Accordingly, the discourses of safe, safer, or unsafe sex are not merely constructed by the interviewees themselves and the particular context (time and place) of their interview but also shaped by the interviewer, the presence of the camera, and then, sometimes much later, by the interpretation of the archivists. Furthermore, they are also constructed by the researcher, in this case me, as I have interrogated the material with certain questions in mind.

The notions of safe, safer, or unsafe sex bring most immediately to mind the sexual interaction between individuals. Do they use condoms, do they exchange bodily fluids? Or do they abstain from sex altogether? However, as the interviews, their framing, and the indexing of them demonstrate, the issue of safe sex encompasses a much larger area than interpersonal behavior. This area includes education, information campaigns, power relations, moral and social values, epidemiology, available medication, the health sector, social welfare, and the legal system. There is a continuum from the individual on a micro level that chooses to use the condom to the macro level where both nation-states and global organizations try to organize safe sex on a larger scale and influence the individual's behavior in sexual situations. In some cases, the distrust of governments' ability or inclination to provide health care led to the standpoint that you have to take care of yourself, like in the two interviews from New York in 1998. In other cases, the problem lies even beyond governments, at a general, abstract ideological level that informs gender relations, which in its turn demands long-term work on several fronts not necessarily having to do with sex and health.

In addition, there is the challenge of not only informing people about safe sexual practices but also changing the way they actually behave. Here, social and moral values play an important role, because of their rhetorical impact. From Kallings's "love carefully" and Eddy the teacher's tirade against Western values to Katarina Lindahl's mentions about Sweden's advantages in relation to the rest of the world, values – modern or traditional – imbue all the interviews. Nonetheless, to influence the decisions people make in a sexual situation is not simply a question of moral or social values:

[S]exuality is intrinsically caught up in unconscious circuits of abandon and denial, desire and resistance. Changes in sexual behavior cannot be forced, they can only be achieved through consent, consent which incorporates change into the very structure of sexual fantasy. Hence the urgent, the desperate need to eroticise information about safe sex, if tens of thousands of more lives are not to be cruelly sacrificed on the twin altars of prudery and homophobia.

(Watney 1987: 129)

Although the quote from Simon Watney's *Policing Desire* above stresses consent as the only way to obtain changes in sexual behavior, it is quite clear, even from the limited number of samples used in this study, that safe or safer sex is a much broader issue than an individual's behavior in relation to another individual. Watney's observation about incorporating "change into the very structure of sexual fantasy" and "the desperate need to eroticise information" aligns itself with the comment from Katarina Lindahl about the need to convince people of the significance of the condom. Moreover, both of these statements address the issue of the intrapsychic sexual script (Gagnon and Simon 2005). How is it possible to make the condom "sexy" or at least a necessary but completely logical part of sexual activity? If this is the change that Watney looked for in 1987, it seems as if it has yet to happen, and might even be described as a sex educator's or public health official's utopian dream, as in the Lindahl interview. However, the notion that safer sexual practices, including condom use, need to become "naturalized" by being incorporated into our sexual fantasies and desires is not unfounded in any way. The societal perception of sexuality as "natural" implies a notion of everything sexually happening with an internal logic, without any artifice. Consequently, for change in behavior to take place, a change in that internal logic needs to happen first. The governmentality of safer sex policies thus relies on the infiltration of the intrapsychic sexual script in order to make it incorporate sexual practices that are less likely to transmit the HIV virus (as well as any other STD).

In the 1988 clip from Australia, as well as in the two 1998 clips from the U.S., focus is rather on the interpersonal script: although the social worker is informing one individual and although the two young men interviewed by Hildebrand in New York also seem to take the individual as the starting point, the focus on responsibility does not really emphasize what any one of these people desire or fantasize about but rather a very pragmatic necessity to inform oneself and protect oneself in interpersonal relations. Particularly since there is nothing outside of that particular interpersonal situation that can protect you – no medication, no government, and no public health care.

The significance of public health policies is underlined in several of the interviews. Kallings brings up the issue in relation to the "dark corners" that Hildebrand asks him to elaborate on. From his perspective, lack of primary health care contributes to the spread of HIV and AIDS on a global scale. Eddie the teacher speaks about inert bureaucracy in the government. The young American men in the interviews from 1998 imply that the government does not do enough in relation to public health, whereas Mechai Viravaidya emphasizes the importance of

Constructions of safe sex 163

public policies in countering the spread of HIV. In 2008, the young physician from Morocco actively speaks out against "ABC-programs" because they do not work, and she expresses the need for a more encompassing and less judgmental approach to sex education. Although sex education and public health policies seem far removed from sexual desires on an individual level, they form part of the cultural and social backdrop of sexuality and thereby influence the cultural scenario that Gagnon and Simon point to as an instrumental part of the sexual script (Gagnon and Simon 2005). The cultural scenario provides a kind of setting and a set of rules that give access to and permission for different sexual behaviors, but it also contributes pieces of information for each individual's intrapsychic and interpersonal script. Nonetheless, neither sex education nor public health policies are enough – a more abstract, socio-ideological level informs gender roles and sexual relations, which in their turn shape the cultural scenario in which sex can take place.

References

Baldwin, Peter (2005). *Disease and Democracy: The State Faces AIDS in the Industrialized World*. Berkeley, CA: University of California Press.
Berkowitz, Richard and Michael Callen (1983). *How to Have Sex in an Epidemic: One Approach* (under the consultation of Joseph Sonnabend, MD). New York: News From the Front Publications.
Bredström, Anna (2008). *Safe Sex, Unsafe Identities: Intersections of "Race," Gender and Sexuality in Swedish HIV/AIDS Policy*. Dissertation. Linköping: Linköpings University.
Foucault, Michel (1990). *The History of Sexuality. Vol. 1, The Will to Knowledge*. Harmondsworth: Penguin.
France, David (2016). *How to Survive a Plague: The Inside Story of How Citizens and Science Tamed AIDS*. Main market ed. London: Picador.
Gagnon, John H. and William Simon (2005). *Sexual Conduct: The Social Sources of Human Sexuality*. 2nd ed. New Brunswick, NJ: AldineTransaction.
Henriksson, Benny and Hasse Ytterberg (1992). "Sweden: The Power of the Moral(istic) Left," in David L. Kirp and Ronald Bayer (eds.), *AIDS in the Industrialized Democracies: Passions, Politics, and Policies*. New Brunswick, NJ: Rutgers University Press, https://ourworldindata.org/hiv-aids, last accessed November 29, 2017; https://timeline.avert.org/?129/AIDS-related-deaths-fall, last accessed November 29, 2017.
Kallings, Lars Olof (2005). *Den yttersta plågan: boken om AIDS*. Stockholm: Norstedt.
Månsson, Sven-Axel and Mats Hilte (1990). *Mellan hopp och förtvivlan – en studie om hiv och homosexualitet*. Lund: Studentlitteratur.
Tibbling, Lita (1987). *AIDS, politik och önsketänkande*. Stockholm: Askelin & Hägglund.
Treichler, Paula A. (1999). *How to Have Theory in an Epidemic: Cultural Chronicles of AIDS*. Durham, NC: Duke University Press.
Watney, Simon (1987). *Policing Desire: Pornography, AIDS, and the Media*. Minneapolis, MN: University of Minnesota Press.

Film clips from the Face of AIDS film archive

Sweden, 1988, Archive ID: 1988_147.
Australia, 1988, Archive ID: 1988_21.
Philippines, 1988, Archive ID: 1988_79.
Philippines, 1988, Archive ID: 1988_68.
U.S.A., 1998, Archive ID: 1998_5_06.
U.S.A., 1998, Archive ID: 1998_34_03.
Thailand, 1998, Archive ID: 1998_10_01.
Thailand, 1998, Archive ID: 1998_13_01.
Sweden, 2008, Archive ID: 2008_109_01.
Bolivia, 2008, Archive ID: 2008_13_01.
Mexico, 2008, Archive ID: 2008_70_01.
Mexico, 2008, Archive ID: 2008_70_02.

11 Sins of the fathers?

Syphilis, HIV/AIDS, and innocent women and children

Elisabet Björklund

Introduction

In the Swedish sex education film *Kärlekslivets offer* ("Love's Victims," Gabriel Alw and Emil A. Lingheim), premiering in Swedish cinemas in 1944, there is a scene in which a young doctor meets a man whose wife has just given birth to a stillborn child. The child, it is said, had been infected with syphilis by its mother, and the doctor decides to talk to the father. The man – who has no idea that he is infected with syphilis – admits with remorse that he once had a casual encounter, and the doctor says with a sigh that it is "unfortunately a very common story." The following scene shows his wife in her hospital bed, looking in despair into the ceiling while saying that she simply cannot understand how such a thing could have happened. A bit later in the film, when its main protagonist, Dr. Bernard, is giving a lecture to a group of nurses, images of children infected with syphilis are shown – babies whose bodies are almost covered with rashes, a close-up of a small hand with syphilitic sores, and images of a child's mouth where the disease has caused damage to the teeth. Through this narrative construction and visual scare tactic, the consequences of an extramarital relationship are made clear to the viewer – not only might it lead to infection with a terrifying disease; it might also eventually affect those who are "innocent" – women and children.

The meaning constructed in these scenes was neither unique to *Kärlekslivets offer* nor to a Swedish discourse on syphilis. In fact, the theme of the cheating married man who spreads the disease to his wife and unborn children was recurring in narratives about syphilis. Most famous among these is probably Norwegian dramatist Henrik Ibsen's play *Gengangere* (*Ghosts*, 1881), in which Osvald Alving suffers from syphilis inherited from his unfaithful father. The theme is also clearly present in early sex education films on venereal diseases. The first U.S.-produced sex education film is probably *Damaged Goods* (Thomas Ricketts, 1914), based on a play with the same name that was an adaption of the French drama *Les Avaries* by Eugène Brieux from 1902. In this film, a man contracts syphilis from a prostitute at his bachelor party and eventually passes it on to his wife, which leads to their child being born with the disease. The film is now lost, but written sources suggest that it also explicitly showed the effect of syphilis on children's bodies (Eberwein 1999: 16–19). Numerous later films would repeat these storylines in different ways as well as the spectacle of babies born with syphilis: "Shots of diseased babies were a staple of venereal disease documentary films, as were revelations to parents in narrative films that a baby's blindness or death was the result of their venereal disease," Robert Eberwein notes in a discussion of the World War II training film *Easy to Get* (1943) (Eberwein 1999: 75). That children are punished for, or suffer from, their fathers' missteps is a discourse with Biblical connotations. In *Ghosts*, Osvald Alving relates how his doctor has told him that "[t]he sins of the fathers are visited upon the children" (Ibsen 2009 [1881]; see also King James Bible Online, Exodus: 20:5–6; Deuteronomy 5:9–10). This allusion was also present in films of much later date. A Canadian exploitation film about venereal disease even made it explicit in its title – *Sins of the Fathers* (Phil Rosen and Richard J. Jarvis) premiered in 1948.

In discussions of cultural constructions of HIV and AIDS, many have pointed out that the discourses around HIV and AIDS build on discourses around earlier diseases, not least syphilis (see e.g. Gilman 1988: 245–272; Johannisson 1990; Sontag 1990; Treichler 1999). In this chapter, my aim is therefore to explore and discuss a particular aspect of this through focusing on representations of women, children, and mother-to-child transmission. Were the meanings produced around women and children in films and other cultural expressions about syphilis transferred to representations in similar media forms in the case of the HIV and AIDS epidemic? As an attempt to begin answering this large and complex question, I analyze two films by Staffan Hildebrand that are available through the Face of AIDS film archive.

The films that I have chosen are *Women and AIDS*, from 1990, shot for the Third German AIDS Conference, in Hamburg, and *Women at the Frontline*, from 2008. Obviously, many other documentaries and unedited footage in the archive portray women and children. My choice of these two documentaries is, however, motivated by the fact that these are the only longer films that explicitly put women at the center, which is not least underlined by their titles. Another film that could have been chosen is *Women at the Frontline of the AIDS Response*, from 2006, but this film has not been included in the analysis as it is significantly shorter than the other two. Also, it is not indexed with any term related to children. None of the finished documentaries in the archive have children as their single focus, but children are a part of both films that I have selected. *Women and AIDS* is indexed with the term "Mother-to-Child Transmission (MTCT)" and the MeSH terms "Child" and "Infectious Disease Transmission, Vertical," while *Women at the Frontline* is indexed with the MeSH term "Child, Orphaned." This indicates that the films bring the issues of women and children together in different ways, which is in focus for my analysis. There are also formal similarities between the films. They are, for instance, equal in length (*Women and AIDS* has a running time of approximately half an hour and *Women at the Frontline* of around twenty-five minutes) and were both made for conference screenings. The films are also relevant to contrast as there is a separation of eighteen years between them. This opens up for comparisons of changes and differences in representational practices and shifting discourses around women and children in relation to HIV and AIDS over the history of the epidemic. The films in the archive are for several reasons not completely comparable with sex education films made about syphilis. For example, they are not fiction films and they are aimed at a very different audience than earlier educational films. The point of the analysis is, however, not to make a detailed comparison between Hildebrand's films and earlier films about syphilis but rather to explore and discuss to what extent similar discourses around women and children were utilized in the era of HIV and AIDS, through a specific case study.

Women, children, and the notion of innocence

As Paula A. Treichler has famously noted, HIV and AIDS not only is an epidemic in medical terms but has also generated a parallel "epidemic of signification" – ever since the disease was first discovered, an excess of meanings has been attributed to it (Treichler 1999). As has been widely discussed, ideas about innocence and guilt are abundant among these meanings and connected to stigmatizing dichotomies of "us" (people belonging to the so-called general population) in opposition to "them" (people belonging to groups who are considered different, "the Others," seen as threatening "us" with the disease, for example gay men, injecting drug users, etc.) (see e.g., Hart 2000: 34–39). Among those who are considered victims of the disease, it has also been discussed how ideas about innocence and guilt are organized along a "victim continuum" in which they have been understood to bear differences in degree of innocence and guilt. Discussing this phenomenon, Kylo-Patrick R. Hart explains:

> On one end of this continuum are completely innocent victims who contract HIV/AIDS entirely through the fault of others, such as infants born to infected mothers, haemophiliacs, and blood transfusion recipients. On the other end of this continuum are guilty victims who contract HIV/AIDS as a result of their own sexual activities, but do not involve in "deviant" practices, such as anal intercourse or drug injection.
>
> (Hart 2000: 39)

Although the categories of women and children are big and heterogeneous, there is reason to examine ideas about them as there are few groups in the Western imagination that have been more strongly connected precisely with ideas about innocence, vulnerability, and victimhood (regarding women especially when connected to children, as in the idea that "women and children" should be prioritized in emergency situations).

That childhood is a state of innocence is a powerful and persistent conception going back to the seventeenth century, and consolidated through art, photography, and other visual media from around the mid-eighteenth century until today (see e.g., Jenks 1996: 73–78; Higonnet 1998: 8–9, 17). Regarding children with HIV or AIDS who have contracted the virus through mother-to-child trans-mission, this conception has probably been further amplified as it can be argued that the human fetus has come to be perceived as the perhaps most innocent of beings. This is an idea that has not least been perpetuated through visual culture, and it has been argued that the second half of the twentieth century saw a par-ticularly noticeable change in fetal representation, for example through the obstetric ultrasound and the spread of Swedish photographer Lennart Nilsson's images of fetuses from the 1960s and onwards. Feminists have argued that this has contributed to constructing the unborn as an autonomous being that must be protected against the interests of the pregnant woman, which is for example evident as Nilsson's images have been much used in antiabortion campaigns (see e.g., Duden 1993: 50–55; Jülich 2018; Petchesky 1987; Stabile 1998). Having been infected during pregnancy or delivery, children born with HIV – similar to those born with syphilis decades earlier – can thus be presumed as clearly being placed at the most innocent end of the "victim continuum." Having said this, it should at the same time be noted that children with HIV also can suffer from stigmatization (Gilman 1988: 267–268).

The category of women is more complex as the innocence of women is closely connected to ideas about good and bad womanhood, especially regarding sexuality. Although the discourse of "sinful fathers" in films about syphilis implies that the guilt in these films was on the husband, it is important to note that many of the venereal disease sex education films had men as their intended audience (not least films made for use in the army). The point of presenting stories in which men's sexual behavior leads to their wives and future babies being infected was thus probably to warn men in the audience of sexual relations with people who might infect them – sex workers or other "loose" women. Eber-wein has argued that the U.S. World War II training films about syphilis clearly constructed women as a threat to men (Eberwein 1999: 82–85), and similar rep-resentations are present in films from other countries as well (see e.g., Koivunen 1996). Although unfaithful men were in many cases identified as having brought disease into their families, this was thus often aligned with a virgin/whore dis-course, in which it was clear who the "original" source of the disease was.

While some women were thus to a large extent seen as guilty of spreading syphilis, women were, however, not given a similarly pivotal role in relation to AIDS. In mid-1982, it was established that women could get HIV through sexual contacts with men, that they could transmit the virus to men, and that children could get HIV from their mothers (Treichler 1999: 47). Nevertheless, there was for a long time great silence about the issue of women in relation to HIV and AIDS, which can be explained by the early construction of the epidemic as a "gay men's disease." Moreover, sex workers were not as central as they had been in relation to syphilis. Even though "hookers" for a period of time were sometimes included in the so-called "4-H Club" – an early expression used to summarize the main groups considered at risk for the new disease (homosexuals, Haitians, "heroin addicts," and hemophiliacs) – sex workers did not remain a dominant risk group as the high incidence of drug use among them made it uncertain whether they were at risk for

HIV infection through their sexual contacts or through injecting drugs (Treichler 1999: 53). Women were thus generally not understood to be the bad guys in the narrative of HIV and AIDS. "To sum this up crudely: when female prostitutes (and other 'promiscuous' women) missed their cue to enter this latest venereal drama, biomedicine gave their role away to homosexual and bisexual men," Treichler writes (Treichler 1999: 45). Interestingly, this was also a discourse in which women and feminists participated. Treichler and Catherine A. Warren have studied articles about women and AIDS in the U.S. press published between 1981 and 1988, demonstrating that not only were the medical press and the major women's magazines neglecting the issue, the alternative and academic feminist press was likewise not giving much attention to the topic (Treichler and Warren 1998). At the end of their article, they write:

> while homosexual and bisexual men stood in for women and were assigned women's historical roles and images, women – including women who were long-time feminists – for the most part stood by and let the men be the whores this time. Breathing deep sighs of relief, perhaps, they accepted for women the much more sympathetic virgin roles: helpmate, caretaker, mother, deceived wife or lover, puzzled daughter, compassionate physician. To this list, we can now add unsullied feminist, complacent about images of women as moral saviors of the nation.
>
> (Treichler and Warren 1998: 115)

Although the discourse around syphilis influenced the discourse around HIV and AIDS, ideas about innocence and guilt were thus also different in comparison with syphilis, which was connected to significant shifts in social and cultural attitudes to gender and sexuality over the course of the twentieth century. Here, Hildebrand's films can be used to further highlight these processes, and perhaps especially as they also have feminist aims.

Women and AIDS

On the Face of AIDS website, the film *Women and AIDS* is presented with these words:

> This production from 1990 debates the worldwide HIV/AIDS situation for women and children. The stigmatization of female sexuality is considered the primary reason of women's particularly exposed situation when it comes to sexually transmitted diseases. In this film female health personnel, social workers and civilians talk about the position of women living with men who inject drugs or sleep with sex workers, and women who themselves are sex workers. Mother-to-child transmission and child prostitution are also subject for discussion. The connection between the AIDS situation for women and children and the active role of male sexuality, is a corner stone in this production.
>
> (Face of AIDS website, "Women and AIDS 1990")

This introductory text clearly positions the film as a production with a feminist perspective. In a comment by Hildebrand on the same page, it is also stated that the film was made at a time when the issue of women and AIDS had not been a central topic at AIDS conferences, which furthermore constructs the film as a pioneering work.

Like many other of Hildebrand's films on HIV and AIDS, *Women and AIDS* is a documentary built around several interviews and a few dramatized scenes. In this film, the interviews are almost exclusively with women, representing different countries in diverse parts the world: the U.S., Kenya, the Philippines, Thailand, Australia, Sweden, Germany, Brazil, France, and Canada. Through the interviews, we meet women who work professionally with HIV and AIDS, like medical doctors and other health personnel and social workers, women who are themselves living with HIV, and activists. In contrast to, for example, *Crossover: The Global Impact of AIDS* (1988), no speaker is used, and there is no instance in which the filmmaker's voice can be heard during the interview scenes. This strategy gives the impression that the women themselves, as a collective, deliver the message of the film – that it is a chorus of women's voices that we hear. The film thus constructs itself as a documentary carried by women, while the meanings produced are of course no less created by the filmmaker's choices than in any other documentary film. Important to note is also that the film is a compilation of interviews made for other documentaries, of which many can be seen in their unedited originals in the archive. The interviews with various women in the film were hence shot with other projects in mind, and are framed differently in other documentaries by Hildebrand. The women in the selected interviews become in this context representatives of women as a group, even though the initial intention behind the interviews might not have been to illustrate this aspect of the HIV and AIDS situation in particular.

The film opens with an image of a classic white sculpture of a nude female figure shown against a black background. The sculpture does not show a complete female body – only the woman's head and shoulders and the upper part of her torso. Over this picture, a number of still images of women from different parts of the world flow past, indicating that the film has a global perspective on the issue presented and aims at a diversified image of women. The sequence is interrupted with short takes of different women experts on HIV and AIDS representing different geographical areas. These brief snippets of interviews underline how women have so far been excluded from the discussion of AIDS and furthermore construct the issue of women and AIDS as a problem related to gender inequality. For example, the first shot shows Dr. Mathilde Krim in New York, who says that "The public still thinks of AIDS unfortunately very much as a gay disease, you know, and it is erroneous of course: it's everybody's disease." Later on, gynecologist Birgitta Gustavii-Koskinen (who is not introduced with her professional title) in Stockholm says, "We have a great silence about sexuality, about the female sexuality. And that is perhaps due to the men's need of control of the women's sexuality." The opening scenes thus confirm the description of

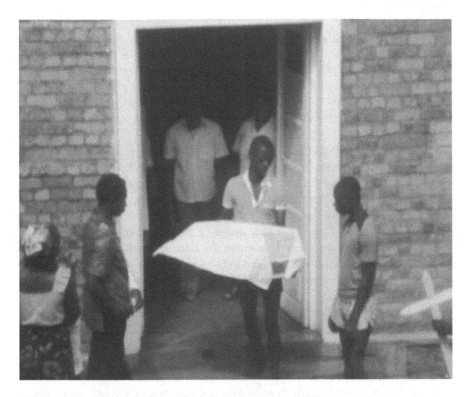

Figure 11.1 Coffin carried out of building. *Women and AIDS.*
Source: Hildebrand, 1990.

the film on the Face of AIDS website – this is a film raising a so-far-neglected issue with a critical view on the power relations between men and women.

After these introductory outtakes of interviews, the documentary is built around longer sequences with women from different parts of the world who tell their stories or comment on the HIV and AIDS situation in their respective contexts. A consistent connection is created between women and children in the film, as children are present together with the women in different ways in almost all of the sequences. Images of children – often close-ups – are used to create emotional effects, but the topic of children is also part of a pessimistic tone in the film about the future development of AIDS. In a sequence about AIDS in Africa, social worker Elizabeth Nguggi in Nairobi talks about how the majority of women with HIV in Africa are of childbearing age. This is followed by shots of a baby being observed by a woman and a man in a white coat (presumably a doctor), followed by images of a small coffin being carried out of a building. Yellow text then states: "Projections for the 90s in Africa: 10 million children born with HIV," creating the feeling that the problem of women with HIV will lead to a great spread of HIV and the tragic death of millions of children, as the women will transmit the virus during pregnancy or delivery. Through the film, we get to meet women who have quite different backgrounds and who have contracted the virus in different ways, but there is consequently a strong connection made between women's health and the health of children. In spite of displaying heterogeneity through its aim to portray women from all over the world, I argue that the film as a whole is thus still in line with a discourse representing women and children in general as innocent victims, and that the film constructs women in stereotypical ways as mothers and caregivers. This, I contend, is observable in a number of ways:

First, it can be noticed through the cases of women living with HIV selected and the stylistic choices made in the scenes depicting these women. For example, the first longer interview is with a woman called Angela Victoria, living in the Bronx, who acquired the virus from her husband. She explains that she did not do any of the things stereotypically associated with people living with HIV – for example leading a promiscuous life or injecting drugs. "I didn't lead any kind of life to get AIDS," she states. In the apartment where the interview is filmed, she is framed together with a small girl who is drinking from her bottle, and she is also seen carrying the girl in her arms in a later shot, choices that identify her as a mother. How exactly her husband got the virus is never explained, but the sequence as a whole suggests that it might be related to drugs, as statistics about the number of IV drug users in the Bronx are communicated to the viewers in large yellow text and through an interview with AIDS activist Jolanda Serrano, who talks about the link between drug use and HIV in New York. Another example is the interview that ends the film. Here we meet a young Canadian woman who contracted the virus from her first boyfriend. Through numerous stylistic choices, the woman is represented as a purely innocent person: The sequence is for example accompanied by a slow piano tune emphasizing the sadness of her story, and in one shot she is sitting at a table with a bouquet of flowers and an open book in front or her, dressed in a girlish way with a white ribbon and bow tie in her hair, and a ring visible on her left-hand finger. Through other scenes, she is also constructed as a responsible, caregiving, and motherly person. She says that she is studying to become a nurse, and in one scene she is shot together with her boyfriend talking to a group of children at a day nursery while her voice-over explains that she does not want to have children of her own because of the risk that she might transmit the virus during pregnancy, but that she has been considering adoption.

Second, the theme of women as caregiving is central in the film. Following the interviews with Angela Victoria and the social worker in New York is a sequence from the children's AIDS clinic in the Bronx. Here, the camera moves through a room in which babies lie in small beds with Winnie-the-Pooh figures above their heads while music connoting sweetness is played on the soundtrack. Close-ups of faces of the babies are also shown, and an older woman with one of the children in her arms is interviewed about her role at the clinic – introducing herself as being part of "the foster grandparent volunteers." After this sequence, Mathilde Krim once again appears. In this interview scene, she gives a statement that is crucial to the film's argument:

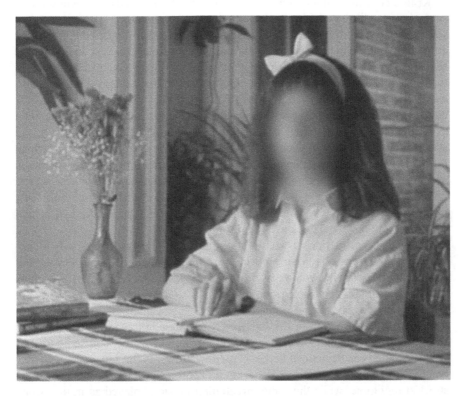

Figure 11.2 Innocence represented. Anonymous woman. *Women and AIDS.*
Source: Hildebrand, 1990.

Women have fantastic resources, you know, I believe that they are not the weaker sex, that they may be the stronger sex [laughter], and that the, they have – instinctually I think – a desire and a wish to, to care for young people, for children, for youth, and for the sick, eh, many of them have training in, in, this, in the professions of social work and nursing and so forth that they have fantastic resources in fact. And many of them have also time as volunteers. Although many women work today professionally, not all of them do and these women who don't can contribute volunteer time. They have a very important role to play in this epidemic, and particularly the one of protecting young people who are sick, from being mistreated, from being abandoned – there have been many cases of families who have abandoned their sons if they found out, because their sons had AIDS, that they were gay, you know, and I think women have to rally against these kinds of attitudes and close ranks and help us fight the disease. There are many ways of doing it.

Krim's statement about women's role in the HIV and AIDS epidemic are in several ways illustrated in other scenes in the documentary, making it a key statement. In fact, it is women as caregivers, educators, protectors, etc. that are emphasized in many of the interviews and illustrating scenes. For example, the sequence directly following Krim's interview portrays a young female doctor working in Rio de Janeiro – Eleonora Quinhalez. In the scenes with Quinhalez, she is not primarily portrayed as a medical expert but rather as a person deeply engaged in helping the boy prostitutes whom she meets through her profession. The AIDS situation in Brazil is explained by Quinhalez as due to the social structure of the country in which bi- and homosexuality are not accepted, which results in gay men living in heterosexual families while simultaneously having a secret sex life and visiting prostituted boys. In the sequence, Quinhalez is seen giving lectures to boys and girls and also taking an HIV test of a boy. Similarly, in a scene from Kenya, a woman is shown as she lectures to a class of school children about how AIDS destroys the immune system.

Third, the construction of women as innocent is also underlined when contrasted to the representation of men in the film. As mentioned, the film is built around interviews with women in different roles, and there are thus not many men at all visible in the film. Among those who are present, however, many are portrayed as the root of the problem. In some cases, men are only shown at a distance. In the scenes from the Bronx, for example, an apartment complex is shot from distorted angles accompanied by threatening music, and some men as well as women can be noticed in the opened windows. In the sequence from Rio, a man is likewise shot from a distance as he approaches a prostituted boy in the street at nighttime, while the same threatening music is played as in the Bronx sequence. There are also men present in the scenes from nightclubs in Manila and Bangkok, shown as they are dancing, drinking, or being in company with sex workers. To be fair, a few young men in the film are portrayed in a positive way, and in a sequence from Paris a number of young men are also given a voice. Here, diverging views are expressed – while one man says that condoms make him feel "less like a man," another man says that he thinks AIDS is a problem of mentality and that there is need for more romance in relationships. Overall, these interviews are, however, exceptional and the total time allotted to them is short. Men are also talked about in a way emphasizing how they are irresponsible and as such a threat to women. In the sequence from Stockholm, two young women discuss the subject of condoms when having one-night stands, as one of them has had casual sex with a young man without using any protection. Here, the importance of always bringing condoms yourself is emphasized, as some young men are said to be thinking mostly of themselves rather than their partners.

Women at the frontline

On a formal level, there are many similarities between *Women and AIDS* and *Women at the Frontline*. The documentaries are constructed in the same way –

they are built around interviews with women but the interviewer himself is absent and no voice-over guides the attention of the spectator. *Women at the Frontline* also aims at a global perspective by giving voice to four women from different parts of the world: Frika Shia Iskandar from Indonesia, Gracia Violeta Ross Quiroga from Bolivia, Toni Ros from Sweden, and Skytt Mykeli Nzambu from Kenya. Another similarity is that *Women at the Frontline* also places women themselves and their stories at the center – only a few men are interviewed in the film. The feminist perspective noticeable in *Women and AIDS* is also clearly present in *Women at the Frontline*, although not as explicitly articulated. The credits present the film as "a documentary on women's role in the global response to HIV/AIDS," and the Face of AIDS website states:

> This is the story of four women living with HIV, who are active in the work against HIV/AIDS in Indonesia, Bolivia, Kenya and Sweden. They tell about their lives and their work with health education, advocacy, and support of women and children. All of these women have chosen to be open with their HIV statuses.
>
> (Face of AIDS website, "Women at the Frontline 2008")

There are, however, also quite many differences between the documentaries. *Women at the Frontline* focuses on four women who are all HIV-positive and – with the exception of Ros – working professionally against the epidemic. There is thus no difference created between experts on the epidemic on the one hand and people living with HIV on the other. The overall tone of the film is also very different. If *Women and AIDS* had been characterized by a sense of threat, not least underlined by the choice of music in some scenes, *Women at the Frontline* is almost throughout a film signaling hope for the future. This is perhaps most clearly communicated through the soundtrack. In the beginning of the film, when the women tell their stories of how they got the virus, a somber tune accompanies the images, but as the film progresses the soundtrack becomes more dominated by music connoting brightness, which, by the very end, shifts to music quite clearly expressing happiness. The difference in tone is expected – between 1990 and 2008 great changes occurred in the treatment of HIV, not least through the introduction of antiretroviral drugs in the mid-1990s, which means that the situation for women living with HIV was, of course, dramatically different in 2008. Even so, the film also points at contemporary problems. For example, in one of the episodes from Bolivia, Ross Quiroga explains the difficult situation for people living with HIV of securing long-term medication.

Concerning the representation of women and children in the film, there are many similarities with *Women and AIDS*. For one thing, innocence is still at the center. The four women that we meet have contracted the virus in different ways: Iskandar got the virus from using drugs, Ross Quiroga as she was raped by two men, Ros from her mother, and Nzambu from her (presumably unfaithful) husband. With the exception of Iskandar, all the women thus became HIV-positive through routes of transmission outside the traditional ideas about risk behaviors. HIV infection is also linked to women's subordination to men in patriarchal societies. This is most clearly articulated in the interviews with Ross Quiroga, who explicitly links HIV infection among women with violence against women and gender norms. In one scene, she explains that men in Bolivia do not think that HIV concerns them. Still, they have sex with other men and subsequently transmit the virus to their wives. About the women, Ross Quiroga says that "[t]he only thing they did to be at risk for HIV is to be married, and the policies, the public policies on HIV, don't target married women," a statement that simultaneously criticizes patriarchal structures, homophobia, and prejudiced public campaigns against HIV.

In similar ways as in *Women and AIDS*, the caretaking role of women is also clearly noticeable in *Women at the Frontline*. A big difference between the films is that children are no longer given the same central part. However, children are still present in the film, especially in the scenes following Skytt Mykeli Nzambu in Kenya. In different sequences, she is seen together with her small daughter – who is HIV-negative – and their relationship is constructed as mutually caring; Nzambu talks to her daughter about not worrying about her mother, and the daughter is told to be a support to her mother by reminding her to take her medicine. The entire film also ends with a shot showing Nzambu and her daughter hugging each other happily. In another sequence, the viewer follows Nzambu in her work with counseling orphaned children with HIV in a slum area. Here, we see her talking to and supporting the children individually as well as playing and singing with them in larger groups. As mentioned earlier, a difference compared to *Women and AIDS* is that all the women portrayed in *Women at the Frontline* are HIV-positive, while the majority are also professionally engaged in the fight against HIV and AIDS. This is an important difference as it means that the women are not victimized to the same extent – they are instead shown to have agency through their engagement. Toni Ros is the only exception, but she is at the same time a different case as she is only eighteen years old. The film, however, emphasizes that she is studying to become an artist, thus constructing her not only as a victim of HIV but as a teenager with ambitions and hope for the future.

However, the agency that the women are shown to have can also function to construct them as role models or ideal HIV/AIDS patients. Here, Iskandar's case is particularly interesting. Iskandar has contracted the virus from using drugs – she thus represents a woman who does not fit the traditional construction of the innocent victim in relation to the disease. However, the film clearly emphasizes the great development that Iskandar has gone through. In one scene, a man called David Gordon who works at the drug rehabilitation center that helped Iskandar, talks about her great journey from "junkie" to "coordinator of a major organization in Thailand." And at the end of the film, we also see her giving a talk to a huge audience at the International AIDS Conference in Toronto. It can thus be argued that, even if Iskandar is not constructed as an innocent victim of HIV, she is a woman who is represented as having compensated for her former sins through engagement and hard work.

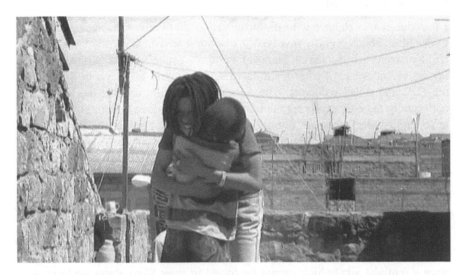

Figure 11.3 Skytt Mykeli Nzambu and her daughter. *Women at the Frontline*.
Source: Hildebrand, 2008.

As already mentioned, one similarity between *Women and AIDS* and *Women at the Frontline* is that they both give voice to women rather than to men. In *Women at the Frontline*, however, the men that do get time to speak are given a somewhat different role than in *Women and AIDS*. Here, we meet two men that support the women – David Gordon and Carlos Ross, Gracia Violeta Ross Quiroga's father, who is also a pastor in her congregation. The interviews with these men fill a function in the film equal to the one of a number of interviews with other persons close to the four main women. For example, we also get to meet Toni Ros's best friend, Sara, and her medical social worker, as well as Nzunga's daughter. These individuals are portrayed as persons important to the different women while at the same time underlining the women's strength and agency, and the sequences are all structured in similar ways, by first letting the woman in focus talk about their relationship and then letting the other person say something about the woman. For example, in the interview with Iskandar she first relates how David Gordon helped her redefine her HIV status from something negative to something positive, and we are then shown an interview with Gordon in which he emphasizes Iskandar's accomplishments. Similarly, Ross Quiroga first talks about her father and we are then shown an interview with him where he talks about his daughter, expressing how he thinks that God is using her and has a plan for her. Although *Women at the Frontline* to some extent constructs men as the bad guys in relation to the epidemic, there are thus also representations of men who are caring and supporting to the women in the film, and who are given an equal status to others supporting the women.

Concluding discussion

I introduced this chapter with the observation that early narratives and educational films about syphilis involved a discourse in which married women and children were constructed as innocent victims of men's illicit sexual behavior, raising the question whether a similar discourse could be found in films about the HIV and AIDS epidemic. The Face of AIDS film archive has offered an opportunity to begin exploring the issue through its unique material of documentaries and unedited footage shot over a long period of time. Using the two films *Women and AIDS* and *Women at the Frontline* as examples of films that put women and children at the center, I have examined how these two categories are being constructed in relation to ideas about innocence.

While it has not been my aim to thoroughly compare films about syphilis with the films in the Face of AIDS film archive – as this would have required a longer discussion of among other things differing contexts of production, distribution, and reception, as well as of changing aesthetic trends through history – one observation that can nevertheless be made is that the films by Staffan Hildebrand have a feminist aim, which cannot be found in most films about syphilis. As I noted in the beginning of this chapter, there is a long tradition of films about syphilis aimed at men that constructed the family as an innocent entity, while placing the blame on women outside this constellation, not least women in sex work. In contrast, women themselves are at the center in Hildebrand's documentaries, and the films are structured around women's voices. Here, it is important also to note that not only does this concern women living with HIV, but women are allowed to speak in a variety of roles – as professionals, activists, volunteers, friends, and relatives. Feminism is explicitly articulated in the films as, for example, many of the women reflect on gender inequalities. Furthermore, women's agency is central in both films, and especially in *Women at the Frontline*, as the work of women is clearly given central space. At the same time, I argue that a basic dichotomy between innocence and guilt is still noticeable in both documentaries, as the type of feminism the films represent involves the construction of women as mothers and caregivers, and as such victims of the disease.

Although it is not as strongly or clearly articulated as in earlier films about syphilis, a division between proper and improper womanhood is thus still present in the films, underlined by the connection being made between women and children. This is most apparent in *Women and AIDS* but can also be seen to some extent in *Women at the Frontline*. Children are without exception represented as completely innocent victims of the disease, and through connecting women with children the innocence of children can be said to spill over to the category of women. Even though this is consistent with existing stereotypes, it is at the same time not self-evident. The theme of mother-to-child transmission could have given rise to representations placing the blame of HIV among children on their mothers, as great responsibility for the health of the unborn is often placed on pregnant women. In Hildebrand's films, however, mothers are not demonized or seen as guilty. Instead, women are understood to be especially well-suited to care for children born with HIV.

Women were for a long time not given much attention in the discourse around HIV and AIDS, and as an early example of a film on the issue *Women and AIDS* thus represents an exception. As such, it was probably part of an important effort to break a silence with severe consequences for women's health. Moreover, as is for example expressed by Ross Quiroga in *Women at the Frontline*, there is still a great need to address the issue of women's subordination to men in patriarchal societies in order to prevent women from being infected with HIV. Many of the women portrayed in the films come across as truly admirable persons with great agency, and as such they cannot be said to be constructed solely as victims. At the same time, the construction of women as innocent in relation to the disease can also contribute to perpetuating destructive gender roles and lead to a stigmatization of women who do not fit into the roles of mothers or caregivers. And, by almost completely expelling men from these documentaries, a division is created between the innocent women of the documentaries that we are positioned to sympathize with, and a mysterious group of absent men who are understood to spread the disease and that women and children must be protected against. Discourses around innocence and victims can be destructive, even when the blame is not explicitly laid on anyone. As Susan Sontag noted in her influential essay on AIDS and its metaphors in 1989: "Victims suggest innocence. And innocence, by the inexorable logic that governs all relational terms, suggests guilt" (Sontag 1990: 99).

References

Duden, Barbara (1993). *Disembodying Women: Perspectives on Pregnancy and the Unborn*. Cambridge, MA, and London: Harvard University Press.

Eberwein, Robert (1999). *Sex Ed: Film, Video, and the Framework of Desire*. New Brunswick, NJ, and London: Rutgers University Press.

Face of AIDS website, "Women and AIDS 1990," https://faceofaids.ki.se/archive/1990-women-and-aids, last accessed November 27, 2017.

Face of AIDS website, "Women at the Frontline 2008," https://faceofaids.ki.se/archive/2008-women-frontline, last accessed November 27, 2017.

Gilman, Sander L. (1988). *Disease and Representation: Images of Illness from Madness to AIDS*. Ithaca, NY: Cornell University Press.

Hart, Kylo-Patrick R. (2000). *The AIDS Movie: Representing a Pandemic in Film and Television*. New York and London and Oxford: Hayworth.

Higonnet, Anne (1998). *Pictures of Innocence: The History and Crisis of Ideal Childhood*. London: Thames and Hudson.

Ibsen, Henrik (2009 [1881]). *Ghosts*, translated by William Archer, www.gutenberg.org/files/8121/8121-h/8121-h.htm.

Jenks, Chris (1996). *Childhood*. London and New York: Routledge.

Johannisson, Karin (1990). "Smittad. Aids och den historiska erfarenheten," in *Medicinens öga: Sjukdom, medicin och samhälle – historiska erfarenheter*. Stockholm: Norstedts.

Jülich, Solveig (2018). "Picturing Abortion Opposition in Sweden – Lennart Nilsson's Early Photographs of Embryos and Fetuses," *Social History of Medicine*, 31(2): 378–307.

King James Bible Online, www.kingjamesbibleonline.org, last accessed November 26, 2017.

Koivunen, Anu (1996). "Syndens spår? Om fördärvets spektakel i finländska syfilisfilmer 1945–1948," *Aura*, 2(4): 49–63.

Petchesky, Rosalind (1987). "Fetal Images: The Power of Visual Culture in the Politics of Reproduction," *Feminist Studies*, 13(2): 263–292.

Sontag, Susan (1990 [1988]). "AIDS and Its Metaphors," in *Illness as Metaphor and AIDS and Its Metaphors*. New York: Picador.

Stabile, Carole. (1998 [1992]). "Shooting the Mother: Fetal Photography and the Politics of Disappearance," in Paula A. Treichler, Lisa Cartwright, and Constance Penley (eds.), *The Visible Woman: Imaging Technologies, Gender, and Science*. New York and London: New York University Press.

Treichler, Paula A. (1999). *How to Have Theory in an Epidemic: Cultural Chronicles of AIDS*. Durham, NC, and London: Duke University Press.

Treichler, Paula A. and Catherine A. Warren (1998). "Maybe Next Year: Feminist Silence and the AIDS Epidemic," in Paula A. Treichler, Lisa Cartwright, and Constance Penley (eds.), *The Visible Woman: Imaging Technologies, Gender, and Science*. New York and London: New York University Press.

Films

Alw, Gabriel and Emil A. Lingheim, *Kärlekslivets offer*, 1944.

Easy to Get, U.S.A., 1943.

Hildebrand, Staffan, *Crossover: The Global Impact of AIDS*, 1988.

Hildebrand, Staffan, *Women and AIDS*, 1990.

Hildebrand, Staffan, *Women at the Frontline*, 2008.

Ricketts, Thomas, *Damaged Goods*, 1914.

Rosen, Phil and Richard J. Jarvis, *Sins of the Fathers*, 1948.

Part IV
Activism and auteurism

12 Archiving AIDS activist video

A conversation with Jim Hubbard

Dagmar Brunow

Since 1987 New York-based experimental filmmaker Jim Hubbard has been involved with AIDS activist video. A decade later he and his colleagues initiated the AIDS Activist Videotape Collection, housed at the New York Public Library (NYPL). Some of the archival footage from the collection has had an afterlife in various documentaries. Among others it has been remediated in Jim Hubbard's own *United in Anger: A History of ACT UP* (2012). Thus, the footage has contributed to creating the audio-visual memory of the AIDS epidemic. Moreover, Hubbard and others have recently embarked on the ACT UP Oral History Project, which includes interviews with members of ACT UP and is administered by the Harvard University Library.

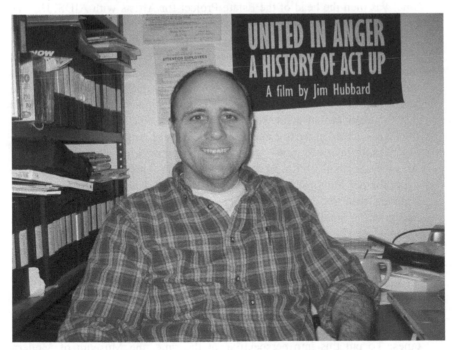

Figure 12.1 Jim Hubbard.

Looking at the Face of AIDS film archive from the perspective of archiving AIDS activist video might help us to better understand the qualities and deficiencies of each archive. The audio-visual memory of AIDS has often centred on the US, not least thanks to the countless activists who dedicated their time to spreading the story of ACT UP and other activist groups.[1] Meanwhile, the Face of AIDS film archive provides narratives from across the globe. At the same time, significant differences exist regarding the industrial mode of production: while AIDS activist video was a collective endeavour, the Face of AIDS film archive goes back to the work of one single director, Staffan Hildebrand, who has been documenting the AIDS epidemic for the last thirty-five years. This conversation will address aspects of archival practice, the impact of digitisation, modes of creating access, the remediation of archival footage and the afterlife of the archive.[2]

Creating an archive of AIDS activist video

DB: You have been involved with the archiving of AIDS activist video since 1995. This was the year when the video collection was donated to the New York Public Library. So, I would like to start by asking you about the when and how of archiving AIDS activist video. What initiated the process of archiving?

JH: The idea for archiving AIDS activist video originated with Patrick Moore, who was then the head of the Estate Project for Artists with AIDS. He was concerned that these incredibly powerful and influential videos were being lost. Some of the makers were dying and their heirs had no idea how to preserve the videos or of their importance. Most of the living videomakers were moving on to other issues and concerns. They were storing their videos in closets or under beds and had neither the capacity nor, in most instances, the knowledge to preserve their videos. The most remarkable aspect of this is that the tapes at that point were no older than a few years old and already they were considered passé and in danger of being forgotten and lost.

I became involved quite by accident. I was working at Anthology Film Archives, a small film museum specializing in American avant-garde and experimental films from 1945–1972. I answered a phone call from Lillian Jimenez, then the director of an organization called Media Network. They had gotten a small grant from the Estate Project to archive AIDS activist video. I quickly disabused her of the notion that Anthology could be a home for the video. We agreed that the best option was for me to study the issue and write a report.

What I found was rather shocking. First, there were very few archives in the United States that could deal with the volume of material. James Wentzy, only one of the videomakers, had 750 tapes including 156 30-minute cable access television shows and hundreds of 2-hour source tapes. To put this into perspective, at the time, the Museum of Modern Art in New York bought two (2) videotapes per year. Second, only a few institutions in the U.S. were interested in collecting AIDS-related material. Only the New York Public Library had the capacity to deal with so much videotape and an interest in AIDS-related (and lesbian and gay-related) material.

DB: How big is the archive? What does it consist of?

JH: This collection consists of over 1,000 hours of completed tapes and unedited camera original by more than 30 individuals and several important collectives. The material in the AIDS Activist Video Collection lives in the Manuscripts and Archives Division of the New York Public Library along with related videotapes from the Testing the Limits Collection and the GMHC [Gay Men's Health Crisis] Collection. The videotapes were made by 30–40 makers, including several collectives with varying memberships. Many of the tapes grew out of the makers' relationship to ACT UP, but the Collection includes numerous independent works and work that came out of smaller AIDS organizations like the Brooklyn AIDS Task Force. The Collection consists of work that explores how the AIDS crisis affected men and women of many communities and concerns. There are tapes about straight Haitians, queer people of color, Latinos in the Bronx, IV drug users, demonstrations of all kinds, in Manhattan, Brooklyn, Washington, DC.

DB: Could you give us some examples?

JH: Sure. *We Care: A video for care providers of people affected by AIDS* (1990) by WAVE (Women's AIDS Video Enterprise) is an extraordinary tape about Black women people with AIDS and their caregivers, which displays a remarkable emotional sophistication despite its evident lack of technological expertise. Juanita Mohammed's *Two Men and a Baby* (1993) is a short tape made for GMHC's Living with AIDS cable access television show about two Black gay men who adopt the HIV-positive son of one of their sisters. *Se Met Ko* (1989) by Patricia Benoit, is a half-hour drama about how HIV/AIDS affects the Haitian community in Brooklyn. *AIDS in the Barrio: Eso no me pasa a mi* (1989) examines the intertwined problems of drugs, poverty and the complex construction of sexuality among Latinos in Philadelphia. It was directed by Peter Biella, Frances Negron and AIDS Film Initiative, edited by Peter Biella and Ivan Drufovka-Restrepo and produced by Alba Martinez and Frances Negron. *Testing the Limits* (1987) by the Testing the Limits Collective, is arguably the first AIDS activist video which detailed the state of the AIDS crisis in New York City and the United States in 1987. The original collective consisted of six members: Jean Carlomusto, Gregg Bordowitz, Sandra Elgear, Robyn Hutt, Hilery Kipnis and David Meieran. *Clean Needles Save Lives* (1991) by Richard Elovich and Gregg Bordowitz focuses on ACT UP's then illegal needle exchange program and the prevention efforts of ADAPT (Association for Drug Abuse and Prevention).

DB: What was the quality of the videos like when you donated them? What immediate measures were undertaken to restore them?

JH: The videotapes were of varying quality and numerous formats. There were VHS, U-matic, Video-8, VHS-C, Hi-8, even 1″ videotape. The tapes had been stored in varying conditions. A few were in climate-controlled storage, but most were in store in New York apartments, which tend to be hot and humid in the summer with intermittent air conditioning and hot and arid in the winter.

Because the tapes were perceived to be in need of immediate remediation, the Estate Project and the NYPL made an unusual arrangement in which the Estate Project raised the money to hire James Wentzy and buy the necessary equipment to re-master as many of the tapes as possible to a more stable format. The Library provided the space for this project. The tapes were re-mastered to Beta SP, the highest quality analog format available at the time.

The industrial context – producing and distributing AIDS activist video.

DB: Let's go back to the practice of AIDS activist video. How and where did the movement start?

JH: AIDS activist video remains one of the most significant cultural developments of the AIDS crisis. The tapes grew out of a large-scale, diverse, unorganized, yet concerted effort by activists and videomakers to respond to the epidemic. They resulted from the widespread availability of high-quality, relatively inexpensive consumer video and a desperate need to convey life-saving information. Many of these tapes, although made solely as timely responses to the crisis, retain an extraordinary vitality. The videomakers clearly positioned themselves in opposition to an unresponsive and often antagonistic government and mainstream media. They eschewed the authoritative voice-over, the removed, dispassionate expert and scapegoating, while embracing a vibrant sexuality and righteous anger.

AIDS activist video is a direct descendant of a rich and varied tradition of alternative cinema. Its antecedents include the work of Dziga Vertov, the New American Cinema, the portapak tapes made by such groups as TVTV and Videofreex, feminist documentaries of the 1960s and 1970s and the political filmmaking collective Newsreel. Like their predecessors, these activists continued the practice of using whatever tools were available to convey their message. In general, they shot on Hi-8 and edited their tapes for little or no money at public access media arts centers, AIDS organizations, schools and, late at night, at commercial facilities.

From 1981, when the syndrome was first recognized, until 1985, when Rock Hudson died, AIDS received scant attention from the mainstream media. The reports that did appear relied on scientific experts to explain the disease, blamed gay men and their promiscuous sexual habits for the disease and sought out innocent victims to pity. These shows were aimed at a presumed "general" public that did not include gay men, lesbians, IV-drug users or people of color.

A handful of AIDS films and videotapes depicting the epidemic from the inside began appearing in 1984. These included Stuart Marshall's *Bright*

Eyes (1984, made for Britain's Channel 4), Tina DeFeliciantonio's *Living with AIDS* (1986), Mark Huestis and Wendy Dallas's *Chuck Solomon: Coming of Age* (1986), Arthur Bressan's, *Buddies* (1985), Barbara Hammer's *Snow Job: The Media Hysteria of AIDS* (1986) and Larry Brose's *An Individual Desires Solution* (1986).

AIDS activist video began in earnest in 1987, at the same time as a sharp increase in political activism. ACT UP formed in early March and held its first demonstration on Wall Street on March 24th. GMHC hired Jean Carlomusto to staff its Audio-Visual Department and the *Living with AIDS* show began regular cable access broadcasts (although a few shows can be dated as early as December 1984). Also in 1987, Testing the Limits began to document the burgeoning AIDS movement. By 1989, ACT UP/New York spawned a videomaking affinity group, Damned Interfering Video Activist Television (DIVA TV) that, within a year, collectively produced three tapes.

From 1988 to 1993, an explosion of AIDS activist video occurred. Hundreds of videotapes were produced. The vast majority of work was made in New York City, although a significant number of videotapes were produced in San Francisco, Los Angeles and Chicago. In addition, there were videomakers in Boston, Philadelphia, Seattle, Washington, D.C. and even Ann Arbor, Michigan and Austin, Texas. More tapes were produced in New York not only because it was epicenter of the disease and the dominant center of activism, but also because there was an infrastructure of support for alternative video. There were art schools and media access centers offering classes and inexpensive access to equipment (New York University, Electronic Arts Intermix, Film/Video Arts, Downtown Community Television), a well-established community of makers, occasional grants from the New York State Council on the Arts and the Jerome Foundation and even a graduate program forging a theoretical underpinning for the endeavor (the Whitney Independent Studies Program).

Beginning in 1994/5, a perceptible decline in production occurred, corresponding with the waning of street activism.[3] One notable exception to this was James Wentzy's *AIDS Community Television*. Wentzy produced over 150 half-hour programs from 1993–1996 and, significantly, maintained his ties to ACT UP throughout.

The immediate impetus for AIDS activist video was the deadly, inadequate government response and the meagre and antagonistic reporting of the U.S. mainstream media. These videomakers felt compelled to tell the story of AIDS from the point of view of people with AIDS. The tapes portrayed PWAs as neither victims nor pariahs, but as empowered activists taking charge of their health in both the political and medical arenas. This was not the whole story, but it served as a necessary counterpoint to the relentlessly negative depiction in the mainstream media.

While AIDS activist video always maintained its critical stance toward the mainstream representation of AIDS, many activist tapes appropriated mass media techniques to convey their message. Numerous tapes employed the language of music videos – quick cutting and the use of dance and rap music to accompany demonstrations. The "talking head" interview imparts authority to the speaker, and thus, substituting PWAs and activists for scientists and doctors asserted the expertise of people actually living with the disease as well as subverting the conventions of the mass media.

The tapes often scrutinized the U.S. mainstream media's representation of AIDS and PWAs and offered an alternative view. Nearly all U.S. mainstream media employed three characters: the white gay man wasting away from AIDS, the innocent victim and the drug abuser of color. From the viewpoint of various communities affected by AIDS, activist video revealed the social, political, economic and medical complexities of the disease. What unifies these tapes is their urgency, passion and belief. Made by members of different communities affected by AIDS, each tape speaks directly to a community in its own language.

Curating online access

DB: Digitising the footage does not automatically imply online access. Legal and ethical restrictions can prevent online access to digitised footage. What challenges did you meet when creating online access to AIDS activist video?

JH: My answer to this must be as a person who lives and works outside of the institutions largely responsible for digitizing AIDS activist video. The answer will as of necessity be anecdotal. Let me cite two examples of large institutions that were committed to the collection and preservation of AIDS activist video, yet remain incapable of conceptualizing and dealing with digital moving images in a fully realized manner that prioritizes access.

First, the New York Public Library. The videotapes in the AIDS Activist Videotapes were donated as physical objects. The makers/donors retained the copyright. The NYPL was eager to re-master the tapes and make access copies. The access copies were VHS tapes and later DVDs that could be viewed on premises. If someone wanted to use the material in a film, a complicated process ensued. First, the re-user would have to view the material on-site and decide what material she wanted, then she would have to get the permission of copyright holder to purchase a copy and use the footage in the new film. Then the re-user would have to arrange for the NYPL to ship the tape to the dub house to make a new tape or digitize the footage onto a hard drive.

Reportedly, a large percentage of the Collection has now been digitized, but the NYPL has not made these digitized versions public either on the internet or even at the Library. This is because they are stymied by the lack of permission. They feel they don't have the right to make these moving images public. They have made no attempt to obtain the right merely to show it. They also have for some unknown reason stopped providing copies for re-purposing.

The ACT UP Oral History Project was born digital. Although the original medium was digital videotape, digital copies on hard drives were made from the beginning. When the archive was sold to Harvard University, Harvard promised to provide internet access to the videos and the transcripts. From the beginning, complete transcripts and video clips were provided to the public on the project's website.[4] Harvard has its own system for providing access to text and images and they are slowly uploading the AUOHP material to this system. Right now, all the transcripts are available, duplicating material available on the AUOHP website.[5]

Remediating archival footage

DB: Speaking of re-purposing, let us briefly talk about the remediation of the archival footage. Can you give example of how it has been reused?

JH: The material from the AIDS activist video Collection has been used in a number of feature-length documentaries including my own film, *United in Anger: A History of ACT UP* (2012), *Fight Back, Fight AIDS: 15 Years of ACT UP* (2002) by James Wentzy, *Larry Kramer in Love & Anger* (2015) by Jean Carlomusto and *Rien n'oblige à répéter l'histoire* (2013) by Stéphane Gérard, many news reports in the United States, Canada and elsewhere.

DB: According to your experience, what is the risk of reusing the footage in new contexts?

JH: There is always the risk that someone will use the footage to make some point that runs counter to the tenets of the AIDS activist movement or the intentions of the maker, but that is the risk that one takes when one puts anything out into the world. To me the importance of making the material available for viewing and re-use far outweighs the possibility of misuse.

Oral history

DB: Meanwhile, in addition to the effort of archiving AIDS activist video, you and others have gathered an impressive number of oral history interviews by survivors, especially those who have appeared in the archived footage, but you also conducted interviews with persons I would call allies to ACT UP. How did this oral history project come about? How many interviews have you gathered, how are they accessible and what are your future plans?

JH: In June 2002, Sarah Schulman was in Los Angeles and heard a radio broadcast commemorating the 20th anniversary of AIDS. The broadcast said, in essence, that at first Americans were afraid of AIDS, but then they got used to it. Sarah called me outraged and we decided that we had to do something about the erasure of the tireless work of thousands of AIDS activists who forced the U.S. government to deal with the AIDS crisis, forced the U.S. mainstream media to cover the crisis in a more humane and understanding manner and forced the pharmaceutical industry to live up to its responsibility to find the drugs that helped ameliorate the disease. America did not get used to AIDS, America was forced to deal with the AIDS crisis. Our solution to this problem of forgotten history was to create the ACT UP Oral History Project, in which we concentrated on ACT UP, the most effective grassroots, direct action political group confronting the AIDS crisis.

The ACT UP Oral History Project consists of 187 interviews of members of ACT UP. The interviews range in length from 1–4 hours. Complete transcripts of the interviews are available on our website www.actuporalhistory.org along with 3–5 minute video clips of each interview. The entire project is now housed at and being preserved by the Harvard University Library in Cambridge, Massachusetts. Transcripts are now on line on the Harvard University Library website http://oasis.lib.harvard.edu/oasis/deliver/~wid00003. The video of all the interviews in their entirety are now being uploaded to Harvard's website and ultimately will be made available to the public, although there is no estimate for when that will occur.

Notes

1 ACT UP was predominantly based in the U.S., although chapters existed in other countries.
2 The interview was conducted via email in September 2017.
3 See ACT UP/New York's timeline at www.actupny.org/documents/capsule-home.html.
4 www.actuporalhistory.org.
5 http://oasis.lib.harvard.edu/oasis/deliver/~wid00003.

13 Documenting the journey from AIDS to HIV on film

Staffan Hildebrand

My name is Staffan Hildebrand and I am a Swedish documentary film producer, based in Stockholm. For more than thirty years, I have been part of a very special and fascinating journey, travelling from AIDS to HIV. With my various cameramen, I have been documenting the human story of HIV and AIDS both globally and over time. The result of my work is the Face of AIDS film archive, since September 2013 owned and curated by Karolinska Institutet University Library in Stockholm.

I would like to start by providing a background to who I am and what I have done in my life before starting to document HIV and AIDS in 1986. After my high school diploma, I got a scholarship from the American Embassy in Stockholm to study student participation in American high schools in five states. This was in the spring of 1968 and there was a revolutionary young mood in the air, a mood of liberal and left-wing change against the conservative and right-wing attitudes prevailing among those who were in power. A result of this mood was the growing protest movement against neocolonialism, racism and the American war in Vietnam. I arrived in New York just a few days after Martin Luther King was killed. I was immediately drawn into the radicalized civil rights movement and the anti-war movement, and I was also drawn into the student movement for free speech and more direct student involvement in U.S. universities. It was an amazing time to be young and rebellious. We wanted something new, a third way between American capitalism and Soviet communism.

At the same time, we were also starting to define our own sexual preferences, in a much freer way than our parent generation had done. They were locked into the traditional gender values, where homosexuality was taboo. During this period, I realized that I was a gay person, and I was open to my closer friends but not to anyone else and not yet to my parents. The first time I met and made friends with openly gay persons was during my visit to New York, in Greenwich Village in the hot summer of 1968. They helped me break down my own self-stigma for being gay. When I returned back to Sweden I wrote my first professional newspaper stories and I also produced my first radio shows, reporting from the American youth scene.

In 1970, I bought a 16mm Beaulieu movie camera and started to practise filmmaking all by myself. I attended no film school. When I was twenty-three years old, in 1971, I was employed as a reporter for the Swedish Broadcasting Corporation and its leading TV news programme *Rapport*, to report from the last years of the Vietnam War. I was based in Bangkok and learned to speak Thai fluently. I stayed in Bangkok about five years as a reporter, a really fascinating time in my life.

After I returned home to Stockholm from my Bangkok assignment, I worked as a reporter for both radio and TV, covering youth issues. In 1983, I made my first full-length feature movie, *G*, a drama about three teenagers in Stockholm and their fears and dreams, about love, sex, loneliness, drugs and rock 'n' roll. That was the first youth movie in Sweden to highlight gay issues. When the movie was released, I had also become open as a gay person in the media.

After the theatrical release of *G*, I made two more movies on youth issues: *Stockholmsnatt* ("Stockholm Night"), about youth gang violence, in 1987 and *Ingen kan älska som vi* ("No one Can Love Like We Do"), in 1988, about a teenage girl and her search for belonging and identity. All three of my movies became box office hits and much discussed in the media in Sweden and they were all based on documentary real-life stories.

But I did not continue to make youth movies. Instead I embarked on a very different road of filmmaking – I started to document the dramatic journey from AIDS to HIV. It started with an assignment to produce a short, twenty-minute

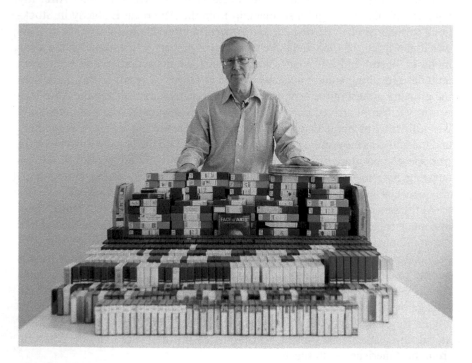

Figure 13.1 Staffan Hildebrand and the Face of AIDS films.
Source: Andreas Alfredsson, 2013.

documentary highlighting a small AIDS meeting with international experts in Stockholm, in collaboration with Karolinska Institutet. This small documentary film project soon evolved into the Face of AIDS film archive. Karolinska Institutet is mostly known for awarding the Nobel Prize in Medicine or Physiology, but their researchers have also made important contributions to the HIV/AIDS research field.

The result of my documentation is around 800 hours of unedited film material and forty-seven documentary film projects on HIV/AIDS, shot in some fifty countries between 1986 and 2017. Most of them are documentary films produced as assignments for the biannual International AIDS Conferences and other related HIV/AIDS events held at leading universities or NGOs worldwide. All this film material belongs to the Face of AIDS film archive and is based at Karolinska Institutet University Library, run by a special team there – Fredrik Persson and Martin Kristenson. You can read their own story about how they developed the film archive in the first chapter of this collection.

At the end of the 1980s, when I started my long journey, we filmed on 16mm celluloid film; in the 1990s we switched to analogue video and then in early 2000 to digital video. Today we just put a very small memory card, looking like a SIM card, into the digital camera, and after shooting each day we transfer the filmed material into a hard drive. The next day, we use the same memory card again to film something else. There is no real original anymore. I miss 16mm filmmaking!

During the making of my first short documentary on AIDS in 1986, I met with Dr Hans Wigzell, immunologist and former president of Karolinska Institutet. Hans was a respected international AIDS scientist, one of the pioneers. He was involved in the planning of the Fourth International AIDS Conference, in Stockholm in July of 1988. I got the assignment to produce the opening film, *Crossover: The Global Impact of AIDS*, to the upcoming AIDS conference, which attracted over 10,000 delegates from more than 100 countries. CNN and MTV broadcasted live from the event. The AIDS conference was a big success for the international AIDS movement and it was the first time that the rapid spread of AIDS in sub-Saharan Africa was highlighted.

Hans and I talked a lot during the production of *Crossover*, and step by step we developed a vision. We felt that it would be very important to document the human story of HIV/AIDS as it evolved globally over time. We decided that the filming should capture scientists, activists, physicians, public health officers, celebrities, and people living with HIV and AIDS. The focus of the filming should be the response to the epidemic, how different societies coped with the emerging new health threat. This would then be the first pandemic captured on film from the early years and hopefully until the end of the pandemic, maybe thirty years into the future. The *Crossover* film project became the real start of developing the Face of AIDS film archive, adding sixty hours of unedited 16mm film material shot in ten countries to the emerging film archive. The baby was born!

A very special memory in producing *Crossover* was when I for the first time in my life filmed a dying AIDS patient. It was in the AIDS ward at the Prince of

Wales Hospital in Sydney, in March 1988. Sydney was also the very first stop in my long journey of filming the epidemic worldwide. This was at the peak of the Australian AIDS epidemic. After New York and San Francisco, Sydney had the largest gay population in the world. More than 20,000 gays were already infected in Sydney when we filmed there in 1988. Thousands were dying. Our patient's name was Lyle Taylor; he was a young writer, thirty-three years old, openly gay and a Sydney AIDS activist. He was just days from dying when he accepted to be interviewed along with his physician John Dwyer.

Lyle, who was very friendly, had Kaposi's sarcoma skin cancer, typical for many AIDS patients at the time, with purple lesions all over his body. He was crystal clear in his mind when I interviewed him. Ten hours after we made the interview, John, his physician, called to my hotel room in Sydney, just before the team would go to dinner. He told me that Lyle died just hours after the interview, which had exhausted him. But he added that Lyle really wanted to do this interview, as his last contribution as an AIDS activist, to help promote future AIDS activism. He wanted his own story to be remembered. The interview had a profound impact on me both as a person and as a filmmaker. After meeting and filming Lyle, I really decided to commit my documentary film talents to contribute to the fight against HIV/AIDS.

When I returned to Australia in 2014, producing the special film *Transmission* for the Twentieth International AIDS Conference, in Melbourne, with 20,000 delegates from all over the world, I revisited John Dwyer. He was then over eighty years old and had become my friend over the years. I filmed him again, when he was looking at the 1988 interview with Lyle on his iPad. He remembered Lyle and the frustration he felt at the time. He could do nothing to cure his young patients and he saw more than 400 young men die, while being their friend, their support and a kind of psychologist for them. Today, John said in the new 2014 interview, the patients living with HIV take one or two pills a day and they live a normal life. A tremendous scientific development has taken place over the years and Dr John Dwyer has been part of that effort.

When I started to document this story in the 1980s, an HIV diagnosis was equal to a death sentence. As illustrated by the Lyle Taylor story, there was no treatment available for the dying young AIDS patients whom I interviewed in many countries. The partners, friends and families of the dying patients therefore started to mobilize against the disease. They became the first wave of AIDS activists from the early years. As a contrast to filming the dying AIDS patients, it was very inspiring and hopeful to document the first wave of AIDS activism that entered the stage around 1986–1988. The international AIDS movement was emerging as a result of their actions.

The activists developed a truly unique alliance with scientists, clinicians, celebrities, opinion makers, writers, artists, youth groups, social workers and others joining hands with people living with HIV and AIDS. It has been very interesting to document when patients and their allies successfully took control over the agenda surrounding the response to the disease for the first time in the history of medicine. They were pushing for more resources from the government and authorities to confront HIV and AIDS in research, prevention, treatment and care. The AIDS movement became immensely successful and functioned as a role model for other patient groups and their allies who confronted other diseases such as breast cancer, heart disease and diabetes.

Another remarkable moment to capture on film was when the big breakthrough of antiretroviral treatment was announced to the world at the Eleventh International AIDS Conference, in Vancouver in July 1996. Without the AIDS movement, this breakthrough would have happened much later. In the first years of ARV treatment, the side effects of the medication were severe. As a patient, you had to take around thirty pills every day according to a strict regimen, most of them against the side effects.

After the introduction of ARV treatment in 1996, the AIDS story changed to a much more optimistic one than before. In the coming years, the disease changed from a deadly one to a chronic one with which you could live a normal life span, if you just adhered strictly to the drug regimen. It has been very interesting to capture on film how the drugs became better and better thanks to the work of the scientists, clinicians and the pharmaceutical industry.

But there was a big problem, the price tag for ARV treatment, bringing new dark clouds to the sky. In the spring of 1998, I filmed one of the first AIDS patients in New York who got the new ARV treatment, the forty-year-old artist John Lessnick. This was for the film project *Global Challenge* for Swedish TV4. I filmed Lessnick when he went to his local pharmacy, which he did every second month. The price tags for his antiretroviral drugs at that visit alone was US$2,600, so his annual costs were about US$20,000. He had to take thirty-five pills every day and had four wristwatches with special alarms to alert him when to take the next pills. After filming John Lessnick in New York, I went with my film team to Phnom Penh, Cambodia, a completely different world.

I remember the shock I felt arriving in Phnom Penh, which in 1998 had an exploding AIDS epidemic with many people dying without receiving any treatment at all. The contrast between the AIDS clinics in New York and Phnom Penh was very scary. I interviewed the young Cambodian AIDS activist Oum Soupheap, thirty years old, who was very angry when he heard about the price tag in the rich countries. In his local AIDS clinic, he had only ten dollars in his budget per patient and year. Soupheap said in the interview that the global community must do something about this deeply unethical situation. Oum Soupheap was part of the second wave of HIV/AIDS activism, which was as successful as the first activist wave in the 1980s. The story with Oum Soupheap can be seen in the film project *Global Challenge* from 1998. The second wave of activism focused on demanding universal access, providing free antiretroviral treatment for all people living with HIV or AIDS. Many experts thought this dream was far too naive to come true at the time. But change really happened, and I have covered the development with my camera.

When I went back to Phnom Penh during my latest visit there in 2015, I filmed Oum Soupheap again. But now, eighteen years later, he had become executive director of Cambodia's largest HIV organization, KHANA, a leading

NGO that has been instrumental in dramatically changing the face of the epidemic in the country. Today, 80 per cent of people living with HIV in Cambodia get free ARV treatment at a local clinic. And the new HIV infections go down every year. Cambodia's goal now is to put an end to the HIV epidemic by around 2020. A real success story, which I have captured on film during many visits to the country. The entire story is highlighted in my film *KHANA: A Success Story*, from 2015, assigned by KHANA.

This success happened because of the global impact from the second wave of AIDS activism. A very important milestone in this part of the history, which was inspiring to film, was announced at the Thirteenth International AIDS Conference, in Durban in July 2000. The activists, scientists and clinicians sat down with the big pharmaceutical industries and the United Nations AIDS Secretariat, UNAIDS, based in Geneva, and other global stakeholders. They made an important agreement which led to the drastic lowering of the prices for ARV treatment targeting low- and middle-income countries that were hard hit by HIV/AIDS. The price went down from US$20,000 per patient and year to first US$600 and later US$300 per patient and year. The leading countries in the Western world, with the U.S.A. as the key contributor, started to contribute to the payment of the ARV treatment that went to the developing countries. At the same time, national HIV plans were adopted in the recipient countries hard hit by HIV/AIDS.

One important film project which strongly stays in my mind was *Frontliners* from 2010. The project was assigned to me by the Southern Africa AIDS Trust in Johannesburg. The focus of this film was different from earlier projects. We were assigned to document the local response to HIV in small rural villages far away from cities in Malawi, Zambia, Zimbabwe, Mozambique and South Africa. We were filming this just when ARV treatment really started to become freely distributed in these small villages. I was very inspired by the commitment and personal dedication which the local activists, nurses, teachers, social workers, youth leaders and groups of people living with HIV manifested and which I was invited to film. This film alone added forty unique hours to the film archive. It has been very important to visit sub-Saharan Africa many times during my long journey, as 75 per cent of all people living with HIV live in that part of Africa. But step by step I have been documenting how the local groups and NGOs have taken the lead in halting the spread of HIV in Africa. When I first started to film HIV/AIDS in Africa, the picture was very bleak and scary. Today, we can look much more optimistically towards a future where an end to HIV might come true.

In my documentation, I have focused a lot on filming young people involved in the response to HIV/AIDS. Several of the films I have produced, which you can see in the list of films below, are focused on young people and their involvement in the response to HIV/AIDS over the years. This interest of mine has a lot to do with the fact that I was so heavily involved in youth issues in Sweden when making my first feature movies, before I embarked on the journey of documenting the human story of HIV/AIDS. I also think that if we are to end HIV in the near future we must listen to the voices of the young.

I will continue to make new documentaries and add more new film material to the Face of AIDS film archive, as long as I have the health and get new assignments. For me as a filmmaker, chronicling this human drama has become a lifetime assignment. Documenting the story for such a long time has also changed me both as a person and as a filmmaker. The unique story of HIV and AIDS has developed into a fascinating human drama during three tumultuous decades, a drama that I have been fortunate enough to document over time on film.

Filmography

A complete list of Staffan Hildebrand's Face of AIDS documentaries 1986–2017, now accessible online via faceofaids.ki.se

Compiled by Staffan Hildebrand

1 *AIDS: Föreställningar om en verklighet* (*AIDS: Perceptions about a Reality*, **1986, 20 min**)

Hildebrand's first AIDS documentary, produced for a seminar at the Grand Hotel in Stockholm, arranged by the Swedish Ministry of Social Affairs and the Institute of Social Studies. Benny Henriksson, who was an important social scientist, was deeply involved in the first wave of activism and died of AIDS in 1995. The name of the seminar and the documentary was "Perceptions about a Reality." Funded by the Swedish Ministry of Social Affairs. (Level 2.)

2 *Crossover: The Global Impact of AIDS* (**1988, short version 27 min, long version 53 min**)

This was the first major international documentary produced for the Face of AIDS film archive. Shot in Sweden, the U.S.A., Australia, Thailand, the Philippines, India, Switzerland, France, Italy, and Brazil, this film project alone added sixty unique unedited hours of 16mm film material to the Face of AIDS film archive. *Crossover* was produced in a fifty-three-minute TV version and one twenty-seven-minute version that was screened at the opening ceremony of the Fourth International AIDS Conference, in Stockholm, July 1988, with more than 10,000 delegates from 100 countries present. The TV version was broadcast by the Discovery Channel USA at prime time on World AIDS Day, December 1, 1988, and by several other broadcasters. The film was narrated by Hollywood actor Martin Sheen and he did the narration for free, as he was deeply involved in the AIDS movement himself. The film was funded by the Ministry of Social Affairs and also by a private documentary producer.

3 *At Risk: Youth and AIDS* (**1989, 15 min**)

Produced as the Opening Film to the Fifth International AIDS Conference, in Montreal in July 1989, with 15,000 delegates from 100 countries attending. It was also screened on Canadian TV during the conference. That film was shot in Kenya, Canada, Thailand, and Brazil. Funded by the government organization International Development Research Canada, IDRC, in Ottawa. (Not available.)

4 *At Risk* (1989, Swedish version, 30 min)

This version is similar as the Montreal version, but three young people from Swedish locations are added to this version of the film. Funded by the Swedish National Agency for Public Health. (Level 3.)

5 *Women and AIDS* (1990, 30 min)

Produced for the Swedish Ministry of Social Affairs and screened as opening film at an international meeting on women and AIDS in Stockholm 1990. Based on archival material from Face of AIDS and a few new interviews, for instance Mathilde Krim, a physician from New York. Krim founded the NGO American Foundation for AIDS Research (AmFar), with Elisabeth Taylor, in 1985, shortly before Rock Hudson died of AIDS in October 1985.

6 *AIDS: The Real Cost* (1993, 28 min)

Produced to the Ninth International AIDS Conference, in Berlin, July 1993, *AIDS: The Real Cost* is about funding and what the real costs of AIDS does to the world economy. This film was produced at a quite depressing moment in the AIDS movement, with still no success reported in the treatment field, no new medications. Funded by the Swedish Ministry of Social Affairs.

7 *AIDS: From Panic to Silence* (1998, 46 min)

Part 1 in an English-language TV series for Swedish TV4. Based on a mix of material from the Face of AIDS film archive and new material shot in the U.S.A., South Africa, Zimbabwe, Uganda, and Thailand. Focusing on the early history of HIV/AIDS in the 1980s until the breakthrough of antiretroviral treatment in 1996. This two-part TV series is one of the major film projects since the start of the documentation in 1986.

8 *AIDS: The Global Challenge* (1998, 49 min)

Part 2 in the TV series for Swedish TV4, on the current status of AIDS just after antiretroviral medication had made its breakthrough but was still only available in rich countries. Shot in several locations in the world: in Sweden, the U.S.A., Cambodia, Thailand, Zimbabwe, France, Russia, South Africa, and Brazil, this two-part TV series added seventy hours of new footage to the Face of AIDS film archive.

9 *XIIIth Cent Gardes Symposium* (2002, 10 min)

Opening film to the AIDS Science Meeting on AIDS in Cent Gardes, France, with 100 participants. Funded by the Cent Bardes Meeting and Merieux Foundation in Paris.

10 *Global Youth Fighting HIV and AIDS* (2004, 13 min)

Opening film for the Fifteenth International AIDS Conference, in Bangkok, July 2004, with 20,000 attending delegates from 100 countries. Focused on young people and shot in Cape Town, Gabarone (Botswana), Kingston (Jamaica), Rayong (Thailand), Stockholm (Sweden), Kiev (Ukraine), and Paris (France). This was an important project, promoting the international awareness of the Face of AIDS film archive and funded by the Swedish Foreign Ministry, which also was a co-sponsor of the conference itself, and the pharmaceutical corporation Merck USA in New York. (Level 3.)

11 *Vi och dom* (2005, 20 min)

Swedish documentary about HIV activist Steve Sjöquist, forty-eight at the time, Noaks Ark and an anonymous woman, twenty-one at the time, Poshitiva Gruppen Väst. Funded by pharmaceutical company MSD Sweden (Merck).

12 *America and AIDS: A 25 Year Perspective* (2007, 24 min)

Anniversary Film on the history of America and AIDS during the first twenty-five years of the epidemic, 1981–2006. All the important leaders, scientists, and also activists in the American AIDS arena were interviewed at length for this film. Especially important for the film was Dr. Anthony Fauci, director of all U.S. research on HIV/AIDS since 1984. He is still, at the time of writing in October 2017, in the same position. He has been Staffan's most important political contact within the U.S. HIV/AIDS arena. Dr. Fauci presented this film at the opening session of the National Institutes of Health (NIH) conference on the first twenty-five years of NIH and AIDS research. The film was funded by the Swedish Marcus and Amalia Wallenberg Foundation.

13 *Women at the Frontline of the AIDS Response* (2006, 12 min)

Opening film to Melinda Gates's session on women and AIDS at the Sixteenth International AIDS Conference, in Toronto, July 2006. Funded by the International AIDS Society.

14 *Standing up for HIV Prevention* (2006, 12 min)

Produced for the Sixteenth International AIDS Conference, in Toronto, July 2006. Shot in the U.S.A., South Africa, Ukraine, Thailand, Cambodia, and

Brazil. Funded by the Swedish Foreign Ministry, which also was a sponsor of the conference itself. (Level 3.)

15 *Women at the Frontline* (2008, 25 min)

Produced for the Seventeenth International AIDS Conference, in Mexico City, August 2008. Funded by the Swedish Foreign Ministry, which also was a co-sponsor of the conference itself. Focused on four young women living with HIV in Indonesia, Bolivia, Kenya, and Sweden.

16 *Frontliners: Communities Leading HIV and AIDS Responses* (2009, 20 min)

Documentary on community support–based treatment, care, and prevention focusing on young people and women. Shot in South Africa, Uganda, Malawi, Zambia, Mozambique, and Zimbabwe. Unique footage from the work in the countryside, far away from any African cities. Funded by the Swedish International AID Agency, SIDA, via SAT Southern Africa Treatment Project in Johannesburg.

17 *From Stigma to Hope: A Report from the Frontline of AIDS* (2011, 37 min)

This documentary was based on the Face of AIDS film archive and new film material shot in South Africa, Zambia, Cambodia, and the U.S.A. The film opened the Harvard University Harvard@30 Inernational Symposium on HIV/AIDS, held in Boston. Two persons interviewed by Hildebrand in the 1980s and 1990s (Paul Volberding from San Francisco and Oum Soupheap from Phnom Penh, Cambodia) were revisited and filmed once more for this documentary. Funded by Harvard University.

18 *Passing on the Torch: Young Leaders in the HIV/AIDS Response* (2012, 24 min)

This documentary was produced for the Nineteenth International AIDS Conference, in Washington, DC, in July 2012. It focused on four young leaders in HIV prevention today, who have been inspired by older role models. The film was shot in Washington, DC, Johannesburg, Cambodia, and Sweden. Funded by the Foreign Ministry of Sweden.

19 *Den längsta resan är inåt – under produktion (The Longest Journey Is the Journey Within: The Film about Steve*, 2012, 22 min)

This is a pre-version of the documentary about the writer and AIDS activist Steve Sjöquist, who was diagnosed with HIV in 1987. Steve was one of the first

Swedish AIDS patients to get the new ARV medication in 1996, and it saved his life. The finished full-length version of the documentary *Den längsta resan, är resan inåt: Filmen om Steve* (*The Longest Journey Is the Journey Within: The Film about Steve*) was released in November 2015.

20 The Longest Journey Is the Journey Within: The Film about Steve (2015, 68 min)

This is a documentary on the pioneering Swedish AIDS activist Steve Sjöquist and his life. Now Steve is a deacon at the Church of Sweden. He was the first Swedish patient to get antiretroviral medication in 1996, just days before he was supposed to die, and it saved his life in a dramatic way. Distributed in DCP format for cinema screening and also with English subtitles. Shot during five years with Steve in Sweden, in Washington, DC, in 2012, and in New York in 2013. The film has been shown at seminars all over Sweden, with either Steve or Staffan or both participating. Funded by the Church of Sweden, the Swedish National Agency for Health and the Pharmaceutical MSD Sweden.

21 Transmission: The Journey from AIDS to HIV (2014, 60 min)

This documentary focuses on the history of HIV and AIDS in two countries: Australia and Cambodia. Based on the Face of AIDS film archive and also on new material shot by Hildebrand and his team in 2013 and 2014 in those two countries. Produced for the Twentieth International AIDS Conference, in Melbourne in July 2014, with 22,000 participants from 100 countries. Funded by Bill Bowtell with three major Australian Philanthropic Foundations in Melbourne. Hildebrand was co-producer and director.

Index

Page numbers in *italics* denote figures.

206   *Index*

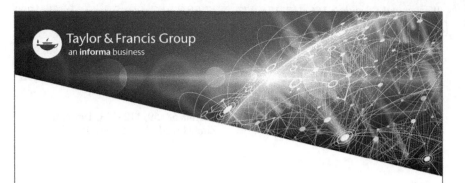

Milton Keynes UK
Ingram Content Group UK Ltd.
UKHW040102071024
449327UK00019B/748